The IEA Health and Welfare Unit
Choice in Welfare No. 30

KU-708-591

Medicine Prices and Innovations:
An International Survey

W. Duncan Reekie

IEA Health and Welfare Unit
London, 1996

First published September 1996

The IEA Health and Welfare Unit
2 Lord North St
London SW1P 3LB

ISBN 0-255 36369-9
ISSN 1362-9565

Front cover graphics from CorelDraw 6.

Typeset by the IEA Health and Welfare Unit
in New Century Schoolbook 10 on 11 point
Printed in Great Britain by
St Edmundsbury Press Ltd
Blenheim Industrial Park, Newmarket Rd
Bury St Edmunds, Suffolk

Contents

		Page
Foreword		iv
The Author		vi
Preface		vi
Acknowledgements		vi
Summary		vii

1. Introduction — 1

2. The Six Countries — 7
Price Regulations and Distribution Channels — 7
i   Denmark — 7
ii   Germany — 9
iii   Netherlands — 10
iv   South Africa — 12
v   United Kingdom — 14
vi   United States — 19

3. Pricing Behaviour, Discounting and Innovation — 23
The Samples and Variables — 23
The Case Studies — 27
Results — 36
Some Implications — 37

4. Discussion — 40
A Comparison with Some Previous Studies — 40
Policy Implications — 41
Towards Rational Attitudes To Prices — 42

Appendix — 46

Tables
Table 1: Six Country Summary
    of Year-on-Year Price Changes — 48
Tables 1A - 1F — 48-50

Table 2: Six Country Summary
    Sub-markets Subject to Price Reductions — 50
Tables 2A - 2F — 50-52

Table 3: Six Country Summary
    of Innovative Pricing Levels — 53
Tables 3A - 3F — 54-59

Figures
Figure 1: Year-on-Year Price Changes-Summary — 60
Figures 1a -1f — 61-62
Figure 2: New Product Pricing Behaviour-Summary — 63
Figures 2a - 2f — 64-65

Foreword

A powerful body of opinion among regulators and policy analysts contends that the development, manufacture and distribution of pharmaceuticals is so different from other products that the normal assumption in favour of competition does not apply. Few would argue that a 'me-too' Ford motor car was a waste because there were already ample Toyotas, Nissans or Rovers to choose from. But it is often argued that me-too medicines serve no useful purpose. Competition, these critics insist, leads to the production of drugs that offer no therapeutic gain over those already on sale.

The logic of this argument is that 'me-too' medicines should not be allowed on the market, a restriction that could be accomplished by widening the responsibility of existing product licensing agencies. At present, they issue licences to products considered to be safe and effective, and the new regulatory expansionists typically aspire to add the new criterion of 'cost-effectiveness'.

Professor Reekie's study is designed to throw light on the merits of this line of reasoning. Does competition yield any benefits at all? Does it help to lower prices? Would restricting the number of products on sale in sub-markets be beneficial for patients? The study concentrates on the economic effects of competition, but there are also strong clinical arguments in favour of a competitive market, not least that all the effects of a medicine are not, and can not, be known at the licensing stage. At that point a product will only have been tried on a few people, and its effects on the wider population and especially on sub-groups such as pregnant women, the elderly and children, are simply not known. By its nature, pre-marketing safety investigation can only be a largely negative process, that of eliminating obviously dangerous substances.

The study asks if there are economic benefits for consumers in allowing market access to all products that pass the safety and efficacy licensing stage. That is, Professor Reekie asks whether permitting rival companies to sell products at their own risk is a better criterion for access to markets than setting up a regulatory authority to issue permission based on a judgement of cost-effectiveness made before a product has been on sale.

He finds significant economic benefits for consumers. In particular, the presence of rival products tends to lower prices. This is quite apart from the difficulty that the price a product can command (and the price that forms part of the calculation of cost-effectiveness) is not—and can not be—known before marketing. Market prices, like clinical effects, only emerge from experience. Moreover, prices vary over time. There is, therefore, no once-for-all price that can rationally be imposed by a regulator on which to base a judgement of cost-effectiveness in an open market.

If regulators artificially restricted access to markets, the likely outcome would be an increase in prices. Once detected, the probable result would be an extension of government price controls. These in turn, would reduce the ability of manufacturers to recoup their R&D costs and lead to a reduction in pharmaceutical innovation.

Professor Reekie's task was not an easy one because the pharmaceutical market is heavily regulated and prices are controlled in many countries. Unravelling the causal effects of competition compared with regulation has, therefore, proved to be complex. The study has used the best source of international prices available, produced by IMS, but the data presented do not (and could not) distinguish between price changes caused, on the one hand, by government regulation and, on the other, by competition. Moreover, the main efforts by governments to affect prices were sporadic during the period studied (as described in the country-by-country survey in Chapter 2). Some of the price reductions reported were undoubtedly the result of regulation, such as the compulsory reductions imposed in the UK in 1993.

Since the aim of the study was to discover whether the presence of competing products is beneficial for patients, the obvious method would have been to compare countries that regulate prices with those that do not. Adoption of this method, however, was not possible because national pharmaceutical markets are not isolated from one another. An increase in price regulation in one country often leads to higher prices in another. The only country with no government price regulation during the period studied was the US and the evidence suggests that prices in the US were higher than they would have been precisely because of regulation elsewhere. Companies must recoup their costs somehow, and if prices are squeezed in Europe, they are more likely to rise in the only place that permits increases. There is, therefore, a degree of truth in the claim that American consumers 'subsidise' innovation in the rest of the world. They reap their reward in having the largest and most innovative industry in the world, by far.

Because of the integration of the world pharmaceutical market, the study sought to examine whether or not there were any detectable advantages of competition within six countries, selected for the very reason that they allow a degree of pricing freedom. The findings suggest, even in the attenuated form that competition is found, that to varying degrees the presence of rival products helps to lower prices.

Professor Reekie concludes that, because of its economic advantages, it would be against the interests of consumers to reduce competition and diminish access to markets, and that policy makers should seek to harness the advantages of competition by encouraging it, rather than impairing it still further.

David G. Green

The Author

Duncan Reekie is E.P. Bradlow Professor of Business Economics at the University of the Witwatersrand in Johannesburg, previously Lecturer and subsequently Reader in Business Economics at the University of Edinburgh, 1969-1983. He held the position of Dean of the Faculty of Commerce in his current university from 1989-1994. Educated at the Universities of Edinburgh and Strathclyde, he has held Visiting Professorships in the USA, Canada, and the UK. A specialist in industrial organisation, he has been published in, among others, *The Economic Journal, The Journal of Industrial Economics, Applied Economics, The South African Journal of Economics* and *The Australian Economic Papers.* He founded, and for ten years edited, the journal *Managerial and Decision Economics.*

In the United Kingdom he served on the Pharmaceutical Industry Working Party of the National Economic Development Committee. In South Africa he was a member of the Commission of Enquiry into the Manner for Providing for Medical Expenses under the Chairmanship of the Right Honourable Justice Melamet. He is currently President of the Economic Society of South Africa.

For the IEA, he has written Hobart Paper 79, *Give Us This Day ...* (1978), (with Hans Otzbrugger) Research Monograph 39, *Competition and Home Medicines* (1985), and Choice in Welfare Series No. 26, *Prescribing the Price of Pharmaceuticals* (1995).

Preface

I am grateful to David Green for suggesting the subject matter of this paper. In addition, he provided invaluable editorial and other assistance Several anonymous referees improved early drafts of this paper, as did Richard Bailey, David Davidovitch, Joel Bobula, Vincent Lawton and Robert Jones. Data collection and processing would have been impossible without the assistance of Harold Hayes, Gavin Johnstone and Pei-Yu Chen. To each of these my thanks. The flaws which remain in this study, needless to say are, of my own making.

W.Duncan Reekie

Acknowledgements

The IEA Health and Welfare Unit acknowledges receipt of a grant from Pharmaceutical Research and Manufacturers of America towards the cost of this study. We particularly thank Richard Bailey, without whose help it would not have been possible to gain access to the comparative international prices on which the study is based.

Summary

The chief purpose of this study is to examine whether there are any economic advantages in allowing entry to markets at the manufacturer's risk and at prices of their choosing. To examine the thesis that there are significant advantages, six countries were chosen for study because they do allow a degree of free access and (varying) degrees of pricing freedom, (the USA, the UK, Denmark, Holland, Germany and South Africa), at least to the extent that new product prices are not directly controlled. In just about every other European market there is direct price control on new products used in the national health care system, which makes it impossible to examine the effect of innovative competition. Yet it is this innovative competition which Joseph Schumpeter claimed to be the 'competition which counts'. Schumpeterian competition is seldom more evident than it is in the pharmaceutical industry. Innovative rivalry is a characteristic feature of the sector.

The key finding of the study is that, in markets where there is some semblance of pricing freedom, competition tends to keep down the price of medicines. Contrary to the claim made by some regulators, rival products serve a useful purpose in containing market prices.

Since innovative rivalry is a *sine qua non* in pharmaceutical markets, this price-depressing competitive influence should be allowed its full effect and not distorted or suppressed by regulation at the level of either the pharmaceutical manufacturer or the retail pharmacist. Rather, patients and prescribers should be empowered further to practice cost-conscious consumption by meaningfully exercising cost-effective demand for medicines. This can be facilitated by information provision, both by a greater reliance on price and by encouraging, not discouraging, sound disease management principles at prescriber, patient and patient-group levels.

Introduction

As a high technology industry, with a continuing ability to deliver innovative medicines, the pharmaceutical sector is a key component in the economic and social welfare of all countries. The contribution of the industry can be measured in many ways, from its level of production to its cross-border trading activities, to its innovative levels and to its propensity to provide high-skill employment as both a high wage and high value-added sector of the economy. Alongside these direct economic contributions to countries where it is a major employer, it plays a leading role in worldwide social progress through its continuing discovery, sale and delivery of new therapies, leading to improved overall health standards.

Various constraints and pressures facing the industry worldwide are making the environment in which it operates markedly tougher. These range from regulatory inflexibility, unpredictability and outmoded controls to a weakening of intellectual property rights. Such pressures are often combined with diverse and inconsistent government policies on price and reimbursement levels by various national authorities. The resulting plethora of different rules and regulations within and between national markets for products which can otherwise trade internationally at low price (medicines are classic low volume/high value products with potentially very low transportation costs relative to price levels) inevitably distorts the workings of the marketplace. Are these distortions worth their cost? Without the distortions, would competitive forces result in products of the quality and quantity which consumers (patients) want and at the prices payers and consumers are prepared to pay?

This paper examines six pharmaceutical markets in three continents: the USA, the UK, Holland, Denmark, Germany and South Africa. It finds that pharmaceutical prices in each market generally tend downwards. Innovative activity tends to accelerate this trend.

Innovations are an important agent of economic rivalry in the industry. This finding contrasts with the view taken by some regulators and some critics of the industry. For instance, Charles Medawar, in his submission to the House of Commons Select Committee on Health,[1] claimed that most innovations are therapeutically unimportant. But he then concluded that pharmaceutical R&D should be performed only in "useful areas ... with a view to therapeutic gain". The economic benefits of R&D, of course, cannot be judged before products have been put on sale *(ex ante* in economic jargon) only the market can reveal such benefits in the light of experience *(ex post)*. It seems at least prudent, however, that scepticism about *ex ante* assessments of scientific or therapeutic advance should also be exercised (until *ex post* judgements are possible). And even if such scepticism were unwarranted, then a trade-off should still be made between the economic benefits of innovative competition and the therapeutic costs (negative or positive) arising from the presence of choice.

Despite that argument, regulators continue to claim that many pharmaceutical products have little or no therapeutic worth. For instance, a recent semi-official publication of the European Commission said this:

> research effort is directed towards those treatments and investigations that have commercial potential rather than those that are actually needed to improve the health of the population. This has led to, for example, high levels of investment in the development of drugs with negligible advantages over those already in use.[2]

Deploying this style of reasoning, some regulators are arguing that access to markets should be confined to those products that offer distinct therapeutic gains.

The counter view is that the criterion for access should be normal market judgement that a private producer is willing to offer a product for sale at its own risk. There are both clinical and economic reasons for this view. Clinically, it is not possible to know everything about all the therapeutic effects of a product in advance. Clinical trials inevitably involve relatively few patients, and so the therapeutic advantages and disadvantages of products for wider populations, especially sub-groups among those suffering from a given condition (such as elderly people or pregnant women) may not emerge. The economic effects of new products (such as reducing prices or encouraging the use of more convenient dosage forms) whether they are clinical advances or not, may also not be obvious at the outset.

The chief purpose of this study is to examine whether there are any economic advantages in allowing entry to markets at the manufacturer's risk and at prices of their choosing. To examine the thesis that there are significant advantages, six countries were chosen for study because they do allow a degree of free access and (varying) degrees of pricing freedom.

The 'price' selected for comparison is the average price for the top five products in each sub-market as it varied year on year. Indices of price weighted according to volume were not used because they tend to conceal the effects of the coming and going of new, rival products. All new products entering sub-markets were studied, and not only NCEs (New Chemical Entities) in order to examine the effects on prices of all new products, including those belittled as 'me-too' products.

The evidence shows that considerable economic advantages for customers result from allowing free access to markets. These advantages would be lost if regulators opted to limit access on grounds other than safety or efficacy.

Furthermore, institutional evolution in the marketplace is reinforcing the competitive pressures of product innovation as novel distribution channels emerge competing not only with each other but imposing further constraints on factory exit prices. Major innovations (sometimes described as "blockbusters") on occasion buck that downward price pattern. Although it is well understood that such new products form only a small proportion of all innovations, they provide substantial therapeutic benefits to patients. In turn they can provide cost savings to health care providers by substituting (less costly) pharmaceuticals for (more costly) hospitalisation or labour intensive patient care. On still other occasions they may provide a cure or relief for previously untreated conditions. Again the benefits are substantial for patients, albeit reimbursers (whether state or private insurers) may now find themselves paying for conditions where previously the costs (in terms of suffering) had been wholly borne by the individuals. Blockbusters notwithstanding, by far the bulk of innovative activity provides economic benefits that impact more widely than a single snapshot of any one patient or group of patients might suggest.

Despite the presence of major therapeutic achievements, or perhaps because of their relative infrequency, or perhaps because of their occasional tendency to shift costs from patients to reimbursers, individual governments, under pressure to contain overall health care costs, have often targeted pharmaceuticals. Drug expenditures are highly visible. As a result, price regulation is not uncommon, even given the fact that drugs account for only a relatively small and often declining proportion of health care spending. In addition some governments, particularly that of the USA, subject to other pressures, have focussed also on the regulation of research and development (R&D) activities, often imposing highly complex, time-consuming licensing procedures on innovation. Still others regulate heavily the industry's distribution mechanism, stifling institutional evolution. They protect a structure of retail pharmacies (perhaps appropriate for the 1930s) by insisting on individual, non-corporate and fragmented ownership of the method of dispensing medicines in the High Street.

These three illustrations of regulatory inconsistency demonstrate some of the perversities which result in the international pharmaceutical marketplace.

Price controls, for example, encourage the practice of parallel importing where basic safety standards are harmonised.[3] In an unregulated situation, where different prices exist between two national markets, international trade or arbitrage tends to remove or correct the differentials. Goods move from low-cost to high-cost countries, lowering prices in the higher priced nation. But where there is regulation-induced parallel trade, as in pharmaceuticals, goods move out of the countries with the lowest (regulation induced) prices to the countries with the higher prices (which tend to be less controlled). Countries with stiff price controls tend also to be those without a strong indigenous pharmaceutical industry, and *vice versa*. Thus, as Professor Patrick Minford put it:

> unlike normal trade in which the country with the low cost producers exports to the country with the high cost producers, in this government-distorted world

the 'parallel trade' goes from the high-cost country where prices are forced to be low to the low-cost country where the prices are allowed to be at economic levels. It is more contorted still: the product so traded comes from the low-cost producers for the most part, since they are the major source for it. Hence we have the strange picture of low-cost products being sold to a high-cost country for unnaturally low prices and then being re-exported back to the low-cost country to take advantage of its higher prices. The net effect of all this is that the low-cost producer sells part of its output to itself at uneconomic prices and wastes resources in two-way transport and distribution in the process.[4]

Quite simply this is government-induced waste.

Second, there are those countries which regulate the new product licensing process so heavily that innovative products are not legally available in the regulated country, but are freely available elsewhere in the world. Until specified tests are carried out, patients in the regulated country are deprived of new products (legally) or must turn to illegal means of acquiring them. Certainly, although necessary, all safety regulations erect barriers to consumption. Certainly all such barriers have to have risk-adjusted cost-benefit appraisals done to estimate (and it can never be more than an estimate) whether the benefits of earlier release of a new product—illnesses curtailed or lives saved—are worth the costs of earlier release—potentially unforeseen side-effects. The evidence suggests[5] that the self-imposed "drug lags" by some governments exceed what is optimal for the countries concerned and have discouraged pharmaceutical innovation expenditures in the world at large, thus again imposing waste on the general, not merely the national, populace.

Third, pharmaceutical prices faced by the final patient (or reimburser) are determined not only by the ex-factory price but by the mark-up in the distribution chain. An ex-factory price may well be competitively influenced by "horizontal" rivalry from either innovative or identical (generic) products from other firms. But final prices are also determined by "vertical" pressures. If some national distribution chains use high mark-up, low volume technology then final prices can vary widely between countries, even if ex-factory prices are identical. Further, even if ex-factory prices fall equally in different countries, dissimilar mark-ups, dispensing fees, tax structures and other distribution on-costs may result in slower rates of overall decline in some countries.

The rate of change of medicine distribution patterns varies largely as a result of country-specific regulation. The regulation can be formal or informal. Thus, as an example of the latter, in the UK an Executive Letter (EL(94)94) was sent from the NHS Executive Headquarters on 8th December 1994 (for expiry only on 8th June 1996) instructing all tiers of NHS management responsible for pharmaceutical purchases down to GP fundholders, that they "must not make commitments to purchase drugs" on "preferential" terms from "companies offering disease management packages". Such packages are part of the Pharmaceutical Benefit Management (PBM) programmes which have evolved in recent years (with resulting downward pressure on final pharmaceutical prices) in the USA.

The reasons given by the NHS for this ban include the detrimental "bypassing of community pharmacy" and the "undermining" of the information required by government to implement its Pharmaceutical Price Regulation Scheme (PPRS). In mid-May 1996 EL(94)94 was superseded by a new consultation document. It allows pilot schemes to go ahead, but is still highly cautious in tone and does not encourage disease management.

Discouraging distribution channel evolution where lower costs could benefit patients and reimbursers is one consequence of centralised attempts to manage the market. It epitomizes the dilemma government faces. Markets are not homogenous, neither within nations nor internationally. Controls can result in price and cost stickiness—perhaps at high levels. They encourage wasteful arbitrage, parallel importation, be it legal or illegal; they have also resulted in illegal but understandable attempts to import and circumvent regulatorily imposed "drug lags". America's provision of a "fast-track"around the regulations for anti-AIDS discoveries is merely an admission that these delays exist—albeit it is an admission made only to one particular patient lobby group.

These examples all suggest that varying national controls operate on the market rather like a pair of hands attempting to squeeze a balloon. Compressing it in one area results in a distortion elsewhere. Despite the varying regulatory pressures, however, competitive pressures tend to be uniform. Furthermore these market pressures are indeed competitive and not monopolistic. The results of the study outlined in the following pages indicate that pharmaceutical firms do behave in a manner which results in competitively determined prices. The implication is that national controls tend to be counterproductive and that governmental policy would be better directed at reducing such controls to some homogeneous, and low, common denominator in order to maximise the net welfare gains a strong pharmaceutical industry can provide.

As a corollary, along with reducing controls on the supply side, government should be encouraging competitive forces by fostering a demand side environment in which innovative competition can flourish. For example permitting or increasing the flow of product information to consumers can encourage disease management programmes and foster patient empowerment.

6

Notes

1 See *Priority Setting in the NHS Drugs Budget*, House of Commons Health Committee, Second Report, Vol. 1, London: HMSO July 1994.

2 Abel-Smith, B. *et al.*, *Choices in Health Policy: An Agenda for the European Union*, Luxembourg: Office for Official Publications of the European Communities, 1995, p. 81.

3 See Reekie, W.D., *Prescribing the Price of Pharmaceuticals*, London: IEA Health and Welfare Unit, Choice in Welfare Series No. 26, 1995. In particular Tables 21, 22 and 23 illustrate 1993 price differentials between differing European countries, the degree of parallel trade and the strictness of pharmaceutical price controls. The stricter the controls, the lower the prices. The lower the prices the greater are the exports intended for parallel importation. Countries with the strongest indigenous industries in terms of innovations and research expenditures are the most susceptible to parallel importation.

4 Minford, P., Preface to Burstall, M.C. and Senior, I.S.T., *Undermining Innovation: Parallel Trade in Prescription Medicines*, London: IEA Health and Welfare Unit, 1992, p.29.

5 Campbell, R.R., *The Drug Lag*, Hoover Institution, Stanford University, 1976; See also *The Patient is Waiting*, a fact sheet produced by PhRMA, Washington DC, 1995.

The Six Countries

The empirical pricing study reported on in Chapter 3 was carried out across six countries. The six were Denmark, Germany, the Netherlands, South Africa, the United Kingdom and the United States. While the six differ in many ways they have in common two features: they are each a location of choice for some or all aspects of pharmaceutical industry R&D, and secondly, they are all countries with (relatively) liberal approaches to price regulation. Or, to put it another way, each is a country with a pharmaceutical industry at risk from further regulation.[1] Since the alternative to regulation is, in practice, competition, each country, therefore, has a pharmaceutical market about which the question should be posed: is further regulation required or are pharmaceutical prices competitively determined?

Before examining that issue, however, it is necessary to provide a brief overview of the levels of regulation which currently exist in the six countries. An abbreviated survey of legal, commercial and other institutional issues is given below.

Price Regulations and Distribution Channels[2]

i *Denmark*

Denmark spends 6.5 per cent of GDP on health care of which some ten per cent is pharmaceutical expenditures.

The state reimburses patients for expenditures on pharmaceuticals (other than over-the-counter—OTC—medicines) by amounts which can range from 100 per cent to 75 per cent, to 50 per cent to zero. Insulin is the only pharmaceutical with 100 per cent reimbursement. On average 50 per cent of medicine costs are covered by out-of-pocket payments. However, about one quarter of the population insures itself privately to cover the bulk of this shortfall in the state reimbursement amount. Copayment, while substantial, is therefore restricted by both the state, and by the population itself. Government has been ambivalent about copayments. Reimbursement for OTC medicines exists only for selected groups such as pensioners. Rescheduling medicines to OTC status, for example, thus removes reimbursement status. In 1989 government introduced a per capita expenditure threshold of 800 Danish Krone per annum before individuals could claim reimbursement. That decision was revoked in 1991 after heavy media criticism.

Denmark operates a reference price system. In essence the concept of reference pricing is simple. Interchangeable products are grouped together by the authorities and a fixed price ceiling (a reference level) is fixed for reimbursement purposes. The reference level is reimbursed irrespective of the actual price of the product prescribed. Any excess has to be paid to the pharmacist out-of-pocket in addition to any other copayment charge which is due.

The Danish reference price system computes the reimbursement price from the average of the two cheapest products in the same group of molecularly identical pharmaceuticals. Reference price schemes of this sort are deemed to allow "free pricing" by manufacturers. The main argument against that claim is that, while companies are free to set prices above the reference price, in practice they are forced to lower prices to the reference level or just below it, otherwise the affected product's sales will slump.

In addition Denmark applied a one year price freeze in 1994 and, in 1995 an across the board price reduction of five per cent for reimbursable products and a two per cent reduction on all others. New products may be launched onto the market at any price provided only that the authorities are notified. They may then be bought by patients with zero reimbursement. The innovating firm must apply for reimbursement scheduling within 30 days. If analogous products are available the classification will be promptly provided. If there are no similar products the reimbursement scheduling may take up to two-three months. The factors taken into account in the scheduling process include the therapeutic importance of the product, its potential for side-effects and misuse, and also the absolute price of the product itself. Thus a high priced product is increasingly unlikely to receive a reimbursement schedule immediately. Furthermore, although individual doctors can apply on behalf of individual patients for a provisional reimbursement classification, government is allegedly "foot dragging" on the scheduling process for innovations. In essence this implies a *de facto* zero reimbursement for up to 18 months with consequential deceleration of market penetration (damaging patients who are having advanced therapy withheld, and damaging corporate cash flow with consequential negative incentives for further innovative expense). Products which have experienced this tardy approach include risperidone, cholesterol-reducing drugs and alendranate.

Little or no innovation can take place in the distribution channel. Ministerial licensing restricts entry into dispensing and retailing. (Denmark has the smallest number of pharmacists per inhabitant in Western Europe. Each pharmacy services over 15,000 people; in Greece the figure is 1,500; and in the UK under 5,000.) Pharmacists hold the exclusive right to dispense and prices are uniform and fixed throughout the country. Pharmacy gross profit is negotiated every 24 months between the Ministry of Health and the Pharmaceutical Association using a formula based on pharmacy purchase price and a variable factor which can be adjusted year-by-year to maintain pharmacy income. The country's 297 pharmacies cannot be owned by corporations (only by pharmacists). Denmark's ex-factory price proportion (before the addition of taxes and distributors' margins) is 55.7 per cent of the final consumer price. The retailer's proportion is 20.2 per cent and wholesalers receive 4.1 per cent (VAT accounts for a further 20.0 per cent.)

ii *Germany*

Germany spends 8.5 per cent of GDP on health care of which some 13 per cent in 1995 was pharmaceutical expenditure. There are no restrictions on the setting up of retail pharmacies, although only qualified pharmacists can do so and they may operate only one outlet. The 21,000 retail outlets employ some 42,800 pharmacists. Final prices are determined by the freely set manufacturer's ex-factory price, plus a legal maximum wholesale mark-up and a legally fixed retail mark-up. Wholesale mark-ups may vary, therefore, and while final prices are uniform, the wholesaler is deemed (on average) to have awarded a five per cent discount to the retailer. This hypothetical discount is "clawed-back" by federal law by the insurance and sickness funds (of which there are around 1,100).

The funds are required by law to reimburse retailers through a reference price system. As in Denmark out-of-pocket payments make up the difference if a specific product has a price above the computed level. Introduced in 1989, the system now covers 60 per cent of all expenditures by sickness funds on medicines. As in Denmark there is a negative list (originally published in 1983) of non-reimbursable products which may still be prescribed and consumed. The German system, however, is stricter than the Danish. The reimbursement price is computed not from the prices of identical molecules but from otherwise analogous products. In other words the comparator products may actually not be therapeutically interchangeable—albeit the classification system may deem them to be therapeutically equivalent. Three reference categories exist: therapeutically equivalent substances, pharmacologically comparable substances and others, particularly combinations, with comparable therapeutic effects. The classification process was slower than anticipated (the aim was 80 per cent of all drugs by 1992). By 1993 the "therapeutically equivalent" category had been mostly classified. Only by the end of 1995 had most products been classified in one of the three groups.

The reference price itself is determined using a complex averaging process which, in the event, resulted in some manufacturers increasing their prices (to reference levels) while, according to Hoffmeyer and McCarthy, "generic drug competition almost collapsed as their prices were also brought into line with reference prices".[3] All products not on the negative list have to be reimbursed. A proposal to have a List of Reimbursable Drugs (i.e. a positive list) has been abandoned. In addition, since 1970, patients make a cost-related copayment for all prescriptions, which, since 1994, has been determined by package size rather than by drug cost.

For the indigent and chronically ill the aggregate copayment in any given year is subject to a cap.

Another factor influencing prices was the Health Care Act, 1993. This required price reductions on all products not covered by reference prices in 1993 and 1994. It also introduced indicative drug budgets for prescribers. If prescribers overrun their collective drug budget (in a given territory or area) the difference is deducted from their income. The budgets are monitored by doctors' own associations. Initially (1993) prescribing volume dropped, perhaps because of the 'squeezed balloon' analogy (see p. 5). GPs allegedly began to refer patients to hospitals to reduce prescribing costs and to avoid being hit by limits on their drug budget, possibly leading to an increase in hospital specialist costs. In 1994 prescription volumes rose, while by 1995 they had returned to 1992 levels.

However, overall drug budgets aside, the system in Germany has been "friendlier" to innovations (which have had to be reimbursed) than the Danish market has been.

As in Denmark, there is a contractual obligation on retailers to use parallel imports if they are cheaper. However, the guaranteed margins provided to retailers act as a financial disincentive to be very strenuous in seeking out cheaper sources of supply. Essentially, the over-traded conventional distribution channel is an obstacle to lowering drug costs. Although sickness funds and insurers are aware of this, there is strong opposition from pharmacists to regulatory liberalisation.

iii *The Netherlands*

Holland spends 8.4 per cent of GDP on health care, of which some ten per cent is pharmaceutical expenditure.

A reference price system like that of Germany exists. Like Denmark and Germany an across-the-board price reduction (of five per cent in 1994) was negotiated in recent years. The "negotiation" was effected to avoid a 15 per cent reduction in the calculation basis for the medicine reimbursement limits. However, it was also hoped that "negotiation" would result in permission to include new innovative medicines in the reimbursement process (at least until the innovation was officially classified as part of a reimbursement "cluster"). This hope failed to be realised and innovations are treated as they are in Denmark, that is, no reimbursement is awarded until a reference price is fixed.

Patients make a copayment of around 20 per cent of costs. Apart from dispensing doctors in rural areas, prescriptions must be filled by pharmacists, who are not restricted as to where they may be established. Unlike Germany (60 pharmacists per 100,000 population) the Netherlands, with over 1400 retail pharmacies (20 pharmacists per 100,000) is not so overtly overtraded. Nevertheless, the retail distribution chain is limited to pharmacy ownership only. Co-operative chains, must also be pharmacy owned, and such pharmacists may not belong to the Royal Netherlands Pharmacy Society whose members may only own one pharmacy.

The reference price is determined from clusters of interchangeable products. Products are deemed "interchangeable" when they have a similar activity, or are used for the same indications, have the same administration route in the human body, are used for patients in the same age category and, finally, there are no differences in the properties across the patient population. The criteria are cumulative, apply across standardised dosages, and the reimbursement amount payable is limited to the average price of the cluster concerned. The "average price" is computed excluding parallel imports and branded generics. However, under the Drug Remuneration System which is applied to the various sick funds, pharmacists can receive one third of any costs they save by dispensing identical products with lower prices. There are thus not only incentives to patients to consume lower priced products to minimise out-of-pocket costs to copayments only, but also to pharmacists to dispense (and purchase) the lowest cost acceptable alternative.

The Netherlands, of course, has long been at the forefront of parallel importation and it is worth recounting that history. In the mid-1970s the psychotropic medicine, Valium, was supplied by Roche (UK) at $1.60, while Roche (Holland) sold to the Dutch market at $1.98, a 24 per cent differential. A Dutch wholesaler, CENTRAFARM purchased large supplies of Valium from the UK and resold the product well below the price of the manufacturer's Netherlands operating subsidiary. The benefits to the consumer were clear. Cost savings to the Sick Fund were obvious. CENTRAFARM widened its product range. Some manufacturers approached the authorities responsible for applying Articles 85 and 86 of the Treaty of Rome to obtain "negative clearance" for the restrictive practice of refusal to supply which would enable them to prevent CENTRAFARM from trading. The EEC authorities refused and instead condoned the reaction of the Dutch government. The latter, far from hampering parallel importation, introduced a published list of prices of parallel imports, thereby effectively introducing a two tier reimbursement system. The concept and practice of parallel imports of identical products in its origins was thus not only condoned but encouraged by government in the importing country. Parallel importers were assisted by the authorities in their attempts to maximise price transparency further to enhance the consumer's ability to take advantage of the competitive process. The point of the CENTRAFARM case is that parallel imports:

(a)   benefited the consumer in the short run
(b)   caused potential material injury to established firms in Holland so
(c)   causing them to adjust their prices in line with those of the parallel importers and so
(d)   also benefiting the consumer in the medium term.

This sequence seems unremarkable, even desirable. However, it ignores two issues. First, (ignoring transport costs) is the arbitrage involved in parallel importing simply pushing prices down towards some competitively appropriate (i.e. otherwise freely determined equilibrium) level? Second, if the answer is no, and the price towards which they are being depressed is below that equilibrium and towards a regulated level, then what will be the long run impact on the selling company's aggregate international operations? Clearly, if the price is being depressed below an R&D expenditure sustaining level, the company will be compelled to cut back on innovative activity and so

(e)   the group company (operating in both the importing and exporting countries) could suffer in the long run, so cutting back on innovative activity and so

(f)   harming the consumer in the long run.

iv *South Africa*

South Africa spends some 8.5 per cent of GDP on health care of which 13.4 per cent is expenditure on pharmaceuticals.

There are two factors underlying the pharmaceutical figure which are concealed by merely glancing at the number. First, the South African health care market is divided into two, a privately funded (medical scheme) market to whose members pharmaceuticals are distributed through conventional prescribers and retail pharmacy outlets. Pharmaceuticals accounts for 29.0 per cent of all expenditures in this market. That market, in turn, accounts for around one third of industry sales by volume and two thirds by value. The state sector purchases drugs through a central tendering body (COMED), the Coordinating Committee for the Provisioning of Medical Supplies. Prices to this sector are heavily cross-subsidised by the higher levels charged in the medical scheme sector. Again the rule of thumb is that COMED purchases one third of the industry's sales by value and two thirds by volume.

The second main characteristic of the market is that pharmaceuticals, representing 29 per cent of private sector health expenditures, are distributed by a cartel which has continuously been able to thwart proposed or actual legislative changes.

In the early 1980s almost all medicines dispensed in South Africa in the private sector passed through a limited number of wholesalers to retail pharmacists. Price competition was rare and advertising of price differentials was prohibited, thus reinforcing its rarity. Furthermore, the Pharmacy Act of 1976 further reinforced the rarity of price competition. Only pharmacists were permitted by law to own shares in bodies corporate or close corporations carrying on the business of a retail pharmacy. Business expansion via normal competitive practices was thus effectively nullified since expansion ultimately requires capital and the retailer could access equity capital only from another qualified pharmacist.

The possibility of new retailing technologies in large-scale multiple outlets (as occurs with, for example, Boots in the UK and Walgreens in the

USA) was effectively barred. Consumers and medical schemes therefore had to pay for a retail structure that offered the worst of all possible worlds, namely high-cost small-scale operations without the benefits of rivalry which would have resulted in a removal of over-trading by competitive evolution towards larger and fewer firms and outlets, offering medicines at lower prices.

The customary mark-ups ultimately paid by medical schemes are 21 per cent on the manufacturer's selling price (by wholesalers) and 50 per cent on the wholesaler's selling price (by retailers) plus a dispensing fee. The irony is that high mark-ups do not imply high profit for pharmacists if their turnover is relatively low and their costs are relatively high. Ex-factory prices, however, lie (after VAT) within a range from 42 per cent to 48 per cent of final consumer price. Because of high on-costs, these are among the lowest anywhere and this is certainly so among the six countries in this study.

In the middle to late 1980s and early 1990s (and probably earlier) the regulatory protection awarded to retail pharmacists appears to have imposed a monopolistic cost on medical schemes. This view is reinforced by international comparisons. Expenditure on medicines as a percentage of total health-care expenditures is far higher in the South African medical schemes movement than elsewhere.

The South African private-sector figure is approximately three times the UK figure of around ten per cent. The difference between South African private-sector and public-sector proportions, however, is of a similar magnitude and although the presence of market imperfections backed by regulatory power is present in the retail pharmacy sector, it is clear that the public sector's monopsony buying power (the tender system) has also played a part in holding down manufacturer's prices in the public relative to the private sector. The distributor mark-ups referred to above are consequently levied on a higher factory exit price in the medical schemes sector. Nevertheless, in a country like South Africa it may well be that the price discrimination between sectors practised by manufacturers produces an outcome where the relatively well-off who are serviced by the medical schemes movement pay more than the indigent population who consume medicine in the State and provincial sectors.

The view that monopolistic mark-ups exist in the private sector, reinforced by regulatory protection (namely the 1976 Pharmacy Act) of existing distribution technologies, is further underscored by the advent of new forms of distribution that have escaped the regulatory net. Whereas in the early 1980s nearly all private-sector sales passed through retail pharmacists, by 1993 this had fallen to 41.33 per cent by value, with 42.89 per cent being paid out to dispensing doctors. High mark-ups have attracted new forms of distribution in pharmacy—such as prescription clearing houses for medical schemes who select Preferred Providers either from the available retailers or from other new entrants such as mail order pharmacists. Competitive forces are at work.

By mid-1996 the Minister of Health had announced an intention to permit corporate ownership of pharmacies. She has also announced that a statutorily enforced dispensing fee will replace mark-ups. If implemented this could spell the death knell of small-turnover pharmacies whilst large-turnover pharmacies could reap enormous returns. This proposal may not have been fully thought through. Further, it remains to be seen how easy it will be in practice for a non-pharmacist to obtain permission to establish a pharmacy even when staffed with professionals.

The Minister also intends to introduce an EDL (Essential Drug List) into the public sector, with case-by-case flexibility to depart from it. This may prove to be little more than a formalisation of existing practice. Parallel imports are also a threat but again the prices in the public sector are so low that the discussion may merely be another round in the continuous bargaining process between the industry and COMED. Conversely it could be the beginnings of state intervention into the marketing practices of the private sector which, apart from the distribution cartel, are relatively free. If they are then it is the Department of Health, not the Competition Board, which is at the fore. The brief description of the industry given here suggests it is Board attention to the regulatorily induced and supported cartel which is most obviously required, not further exercises of monopsony Departmental buying power.

v *United Kingdom*

The UK spends 6.8 per cent of GDP on health care and 11.0 per cent of that is accounted for by pharmaceutical expenditures.

The NHS as a monopsonist attempts to control expenditures on pharmaceuticals in a variety of ways. First, consumption by patients is notionally affected by the prescription charge. Second, it influences prescribing patterns by doctors by laying down guidelines and also (in limited areas) rules on what can and cannot, and on what should and should not, be prescribed. Finally, it attempts to influence prices directly at manufacturer level.

Pharmaceutical manufacturers supplying the NHS are subject to the Pharmaceutical Price Regulation Scheme (PPRS) which is a non-statutory agreement between the industry and the Department of Health. Despite its name, the scheme aims to control profits rather than prices. A company is assigned a rate of return on assets which is based on an overall figure for the industry but which takes account of its particular circumstances, especially its economic contribution, realized and potential, in terms of capital investment, research expenditures, employment and foreign earnings. The scheme, which may be traced back to 1957, has recently been renegotiated and a revised version came into effect on 1st October 1993. Essentially the PPRS limits the amount of profit a company can earn on its total sales of branded products to the NHS. If profits rise above a specified figure, product price reductions may be required and, if profits fall below an agreed level, price increases may be permitted. The initial price of a new product is not controlled.

Green and Lucas assert that the "heart of the system is the annual financial return (AFR)".[4] The AFR must distinguish between sales to the NHS and other business. Production costs must be apportioned between NHS and export business. Capital must be valued at historic cost, and transfer prices (the charges made for supplies obtained from overseas affiliates) disclosed or imputed by the Department of Health. From the AFR decisions are taken as to whether the firm's return on assets is reasonable. Research and development costs are set by the Department of Health as a percentage of sales to the NHS (20 per cent for the industry as a whole).

"Reasonableness" is a concept with no generally accepted meaning. Officially, the reasonableness of the return on capital earned by companies on home sales of NHS medicines is a matter for negotiation within a published range between companies and the Department of Health. Under the current scheme (and since 1988) the industry and government have tried to remove the target rate of return from the debating arena by agreeing on a figure which will take account of "any relevant and significant alterations since the last PPRS rate change in the underlying average return on capital of British Industry as brought out for example in relevant changes in the FT 500 index or of any relevant policies that may be generally in force on the appropriate levels of profitability on public sector business".

The current "headline figure" for negotiations is a band of 17-21 per cent. Whether movements in this average accounting return on capital in British industry should be "reasonably" correlated with that of the pharmaceutical industry, begs the question.

In addition, companies may in certain circumstances be permitted to retain profit above their target range. This discretionary allowance (previously called the "grey area" and now the "margin of tolerance") has varied. Under the 1986 scheme, companies could retain profits if they did not exceed 50 per cent of the agreed targets. The Department could allow such retention of profits if they arose from: "the launch of a new product, improved efficiency or other factors clearly arising from the company's own efforts". Under the 1993 scheme, companies have an automatic right to retain profits within the margin of tolerance of 25 per cent above target. If company profits fall below target, they have no right to seek a price increase unless profits are more than 25 per cent below target.

As a consequence of negotiations leading up to the 1993 Scheme now in place, an immediate general across-the-board price reduction of 2.5 per cent on all branded products was implemented, followed by three years of price restraint.[5]

In addition to price controls imposed through the PPRS, the NHS deploys other methods of limiting expenditure on pharmaceuticals. The methods include cash limits, target budgets (known as "indicative prescribing amounts" until April 1994), the Selected List, prescription charges and controls on the volume of advertising allowed for profit calculation purposes in PPRS discussions. Cash limits apply to fundholding General Practitioners only. Since the introduction of the fundholding scheme in 1991 the number of fundholders has grown to well over 10,000 GPs. Their practices cover approximately 50 per cent of the population, and it is probable that this percentage will continue to increase.

It is worth looking more closely at fundholding practices since they are both a new phenomenon and their prescribing incentives differ somewhat from the conventional practices in the NHS. Fundholders receive cash limited budgets which can be allocated for certain defined purchases (including pharmaceuticals) on behalf of their patients. The budgets are approved and distributed directly and annually by the NHS Executive (NHSE) Regional Office (of which there are eight in England). A fundholder who overshoots his cash limit cannot continue to supply unless other monetary arrangements are made with NHS approval. Alternatively at year end any cash surplus can be appropriated by the fundholder for approved practice purposes. The incentives in place are therefore not to overspend but to conserve resources and utilise the cash budget cost effectively.

Pharmaceuticals represent only one item in the fundholder's portfolio of expenditure items and the verdict on fundholding prescribing behaviour has still to come in. However, the Audit Commission[6] indicated that the first results were encouraging. During 1992/93, for example, fundholders achieved average expenditure levels on pharmaceuticals 9.4 per cent less per surveyed prescribing unit than those of other practices. Further, the growth rate of expenditures by fundholding practices ranged from 2.0 to 4.3 per cent less per annum than the 12 per cent rate of increase of non-fundholders. In its most recent report[7] the Commission provides data confirming this evidence but which cautions against expecting expenditures on drugs forever and for always to either be less or to grow less among one sub-set of purchasers or prescribers. In 1993/94 expenditures on prescribing were less on average among all fundholders vis-a-vis non-fundholders, but only with the earliest practices to opt for fundholding (Wave 1) was the difference statistically significant. Wave 1 fundholders would, presumably be the most commercially aggressive groups since they were the first to self-select into the system. On the other hand diminishing returns from savings have now apparently set in for the Wave 1 group. Fundholders of all vintages again had a rate of increase in prescribing expenditures below the non-fundholding average, but only among the most recent group (Wave 3) was that slower rate of increase statistically significant. The law of diminishing returns has not been repealed. Whether its impact has been felt surprisingly quickly—or not—is another issue. The fundholder, after all, is not only under an incentive to conserve costs but, like any other pre-payment system, there is an incentive to underspend. Only when the cash nexus is direct between patient and provider is it possible in principle to avoid moral hazard of this sort altogether. The prescription charge of £5.25 does not achieve this cash nexus even for pharmaceuticals since 88 per cent of scripts written are exempt from even this modest copayment.

During the period of the study there were some 90 Family Health Services Authorities (FHSAs) in England.[8] Each FHSA had a chief executive responsible for allocating and monitoring cash limited GP fundholder budgets and for financing and monitoring the budgets for the remaining majority of GPs for the indicative prescribing scheme. The FHSA was required to monitor GP prescribing and then to initiate early and effective action of any "excessive prescribing" defined as significant divergence of actual expenditures from that planned or predicted. GPs have limited clinical freedom to treat patients according to their professional discretion. For example they were expected to stay within the "indicative drug amount" ("target budget" from April 1994) set by the FHSA. The Audit Commission found that 85 per cent of practices (92 per cent of larger practices) overspent these amounts in 1991/92.[9] The total overshoot was 7.5 per cent of the budgeted amount. In setting indicative amounts FHSAs considered practices' historic spending patterns, comparable average costs for the FHSA, the special circumstances of the practice including high cost patients, anticipated changes in demand and an allowance for the forecast increase in the cost of drugs. (For fundholders, the prescribing costs are actual allocations financed from the overall drug budgets allocated to the NHSE regional office.)

The "indicative drug amount" is not cash limited but corrective actions, such as withholding of remuneration, may be taken against prescribers who persistently overspend the set level. Each FHSA had a prescribing medical adviser who, *inter alia*, provided expert advice to the FHSA on the drawing up of prescribing profiles for each practice, the setting of amounts for individual practices and the monitoring of practices' performance. Since August 1988 the prescribing patterns and costs of every GP have been monitored by an information system known as PACT (Prescription Analysis and Cost). From 1991 each GP received a monthly budget statement of practice expenditure and indicative amounts. In addition prescribing costs of a practice compared with local and national patterns and with practice data from the previous year are provided. The availability of drugs where generic prescribing would reduce costs is also indicated.

Another route followed by government to exert downward pressure on pharmaceutical expenditures is the Selected List. First introduced in April 1985, this meant that fewer drugs were available on prescription under the NHS. Specifically seven drug categories were nominated: minor pain killers, cough and cold remedies, laxatives, indigestion remedies, vitamins and tonics and sedatives. A selected list of around 400 products in these categories were duly excluded. The objectives were to encourage purchase from chemists over-the-counter and without prescription. The "blacklisting" was not unsuccessful as measured by some yardsticks. For example, according to the Office of Health Economics, expectorants and cough suppressants—the second most commonly prescribed sub-grouping in 1970—had fallen to the nineteenth ranking by 1990. A further ten categories were announced in late 1992, some more products have subsequently been blacklisted and in other cases product prices have been reduced in order to remove the threat of listing. The Selected List thus not only proscribes prescription of nominated products but removes the previously available blanket pricing "freedom" under the PPRS for the unlisted, and so tacitly approved products in the seventeen categories concerned.

Government has also devoted substantial efforts towards promoting greater generic prescribing. As a result the proportion of prescriptions dispensed in generic forms grew appreciably to account for over 40 per cent of the total number of prescriptions dispensed by chemists, as compared with 25 per cent in 1985.

The Department of Health actively encourages dispensing chemists to purchase parallel imports rather than domestically produced equivalents. From 1991 the chemist had been allowed to retain the full difference between the official list or reimbursement price and the price he paid for the parallel product. If the individual pharmacist fails to react to this incentive he will lose some of it anyway when the Department of Health "claws it back" in subsequent remuneration awards made 12-24 months later. These are computed on the assumption that the parallel imports observed in aggregate by government through its licensing and statistical trade records are distributed through the retail industry as a whole.

In the UK retail and other distribution margins are low. Ex-factory prices account for 87.5 per cent of total costs. Medicines are VAT exempt and distributors margins and fees (wholesale and retail) account for the remaining 12.5 per cent. Partly this reflects the monopsony power exercised by the NHS on the remuneration of pharmacists. Partly it reflects the fact that multiple chain pharmacy operations in the United Kingdom are not uncommon and hence scale economies can be reaped. More patients can be served per pharmacy and also professional staff themselves can be used more productively. Chain store ownership (and hence larger unit pharmacies) are epitomised by the statistics showing that the UK had 14,620 pharmacies in 1962 and 12,300 in 1994. With only 21 pharmacists per 100,000 population (Germany has 60 as does the USA) the UK has one of the lowest ratios of pharmacists to population among the OECD countries. The improving productivity of retail pharmacists can be seen from the rise in prescription numbers dispensed. In 1984 each UK chemist handled 33,752 prescription items. This had risen to 42,343 per annum in 1994, an increase of over 25 per cent.

vi *United States*

The USA spends 14.5 per cent of GDP on health costs of which 5.6 per cent is directed at outpatient pharmaceutical expenditures.

Of the six countries examined here it has the most pluralistic and decentralised health care market (even ahead of South Africa). Twenty two per cent of the population are covered by the government schemes for the elderly or indigent, Medicare and Medicaid, 62 per cent have private insurance coverage while 15 per cent are uninsured. In 1970, 90 per cent of all expenditures on medicines were out-of-pocket. This had fallen by 1995 to 42 per cent, still well above the average copayment levels in any of the other five countries. (Although this possibly understates the average level of copayment since 25 per cent of the population have no coverage at all for prescription drugs). The decline in out-of-pocket payments for drugs is partly due to the increasing sophistication of the various insurers. Third party reimbursers have evolved over the last few years as powerful and sophisticated buyers of health care inputs, including pharmaceuticals. While substantial copayments remain as disincentives to over utilisation, patients and premium providers have chosen to include drugs in their package of coverage in the belief that the third party buyer can make a more cost-effective purchase on their behalf than they can themselves.

Legislative barriers to the growth of Health Maintenance Organisations (HMOs) have crumbled. As a consequence managed care has grown rapidly. HMOs increasingly rely on drug utilisation reviews, limited formularies, generic substitution and step therapy.

Initially (after 1980 according to Burstall)[10] the widespread use of generics resulted in drug prices rising on average. The paradox is explained by the relatively higher increases in price levied on patent protected and new products. Continued competition between manufacturers and pressure from distributors and reimbursers, however, ensured that this was merely a temporary reaction as the players in the marketplace continued to adjust to new and additional pressures.

A study by the Boston Consulting Group[11] showed how discounts on consumer prices paid for pharmaceuticals had risen from four per cent to 14 per cent between 1987 and 1992 (on a weighted average basis). This rise in discounting was parallelled by declines in the importance of conventional links in the distribution chain where discounting had been low or non-existent. Traditional retail pharmacy's share of the total market fell from 35 to 25 per cent. Managed retail pharmacies, however, (that is chains, HMO pharmacists, and preferred providers) grew in importance from 20 to 35 per cent of the market (offering discounts of 25 per cent, up from 10 per cent in 1987). Mail order pharmacies increased their discounts over the period from 15 to 30 per cent (and their market share grew from an insignificant level to five per cent). Managed hospital pharmacies similarly displaced traditional hospital pharmacies, and offered substantially higher discounts.

While this was occurring in the private sector the state sector has also been able to move in lock-step with the trend to increasing price consciousness. For example, Medicaid reimbursed pharmacists at average wholesale price (AWP) plus a dispensing fee. If pharmacy purchasers negotiate discounts off AWP with the wholesalers, they could be more competitive on the dispensing fee for Medicaid prescriptions. Now, state and federal legislation is intending to set reimbursement rates at AWP minus a discount, plus a dispensing fee for filling prescriptions. Medicaid programmes also receive rebates, based on the average manufacturer's price. Legislation requires drug manufacturers to pay rebates to the level of the "most favoured purchaser" in the marketplace. The "most favoured purchaser" refers to the purchasers that receive the best national price for pharmaceutical products, typically hospitals and managed care entities. The rebates are based on pharmacy usage data and determined by a national formula applied across the country. The Medicaid rebates affect generic firms more leniently than brand-name firms. But, of course, while the rebate is smaller for generic products, so are the net prices. At the same time as government and private reimbursers are exercising downward pressure on price both at the factory gate and to the final payer, a new type of enterprise designed to cut and contain costs has emerged. These innovative newcomers to the distribution channel are the PBMs or Pharmaceutical Benefit Managers. They are most obvious in the USA and some are trying to emerge in South Africa.

The proximate business purpose of PBMs was to cut the costs of health insurers (insurance companies, HMOs, and large employers) caused by high prices at the factory gate or in the distribution chain. A PBM offers the insurer the chance to cut costs by taking over the responsibility for the supply of medication, either for all diseases or for selected ones, at a substantially lower cost than under existing arrangements. The PBM is able to do this by negotiating discounts from manufacturers and from the wholesale and pharmacy links in the distribution chain, usually contracting with a sub-set of pharmacies to supply the needs of the PBM client. A small percentage of medicines, often in more rural areas, is distributed through the mail from specialised pharmacies. Variations on this theme have developed, for example by widening the focus from pharmaceutical to the broader management of a disease bringing in non-pharmaceutical interventions; and by bringing pharmacies into the arrangements on a contracted basis.

More recently PBMs (and some HMOs) have developed computer systems which enable them to monitor the use of drugs and build up patient profiles. Access to these data enables companies to widen the focus of their operations and develop the concept of disease management, including both pharmaceutical and non-pharmaceutical interventions (sometimes known as TDM, Total Disease Management, or alternatively integrated health care). As was noted earlier TDM schemes were for a time informally "outlawed" and are still not encouraged by the NHS in the UK.

PBMs have rapidly come to account for more than a quarter of all medicines sold in the US, covering some 50 million insured Americans. They therefore pose a serious threat to the existence of wholesalers and traditional retail pharmacies. Some pharmaceutical manufacturers have spotted a possible further opportunity and are buying into PBMs in order to introduce and encourage the integrated health care concept—as well as to attempt to alleviate the threat from yet another source of competitive pressure in the pharmaceutical marketplace. SmithKline/Beecham, Eli Lilly and Merck have all done this. The new combined companies have considered how to export the PBM concept to other countries. Independent PBMs in the US are also considering whether there are ways they can enter foreign markets (for example, by selling prescribing support, information technology systems). To date, however, very little has actually been implemented.

Conclusion

The six countries have different regulatory systems, varying in the intensity with which prices are controlled by law. The alternative in practice to price regulation by legal restraint is price levels determined by competition. Prices so arrived at reflect the values placed on the product by consumers, and if willingly paid and accepted, the full costs incurred by producers. If the varying regulations by country are effective one would expect to find differing pricing patterns evolving. If competitive forces are relatively strong, however, (that is relative to regulation) one would anticipate similar pricing patterns to be displayed across countries. (And while regulations may differ, pharmaceutical producers and consumers are remarkably similar. It is their values and their costs which enter into freely determined demand and supply patterns, not the values or costs of others.)

The pricing patterns revealed below suggest competitive forces are far from repressed. The question must then be posed: why not permit the price depressing influence of competition its full effect? Why distort or suppress competition by regulation at the level of the manufacturer or the retailer? Why not encourage it by enhancing information flows to prescribers and patients? This is further elaborated in Chapter 4. First, Chapter 3 reports on the results of the study.

Notes

1 For example, in the United Kingdom the Pharmaceutical Price Regulation Scheme may be amended after the election pending in 1996 or 1997. In South Africa a Pricing Committee to monitor and approve medicine price levels was proposed in early 1996.

2 Information and data in this section were compiled from the following sources: a) *Facts 1995* MEFA Copenhagen, 199; b) *Compendium of Health Statistics*, London: Office of Health Economics, 1995; c) Hoffmeyer, U. and McCarthy, T.R., *Financing Health Care*, Dordrecht: Clair Academic Publishers, 1995; d) Reekie, W.D., *Health Care Options for South Africa: Lessons from the UK and USA*, Johannesburg: Free Market Foundation, 1995; e) *Annual Report 1994*, Nefarma, Utrecht.

3 Hoffmeyer and McCarthy, *op. cit.,* 1995, p. 465.

4 Green, D.G. and Lucas, D.A., *Medicard: A Better Way to Pay for Medicines?* Choice in Welfare Series No. 26, London: IEA Health and Welfare Unit, 1993.

5 Companies were required to add to their actual PPRS profit the notional profit loss resulting from the 2.5 per cent price cut of 1993. The result is that their PPRS profit is higher than the true figure so that companies are far less likely to fall below the bottom of the margin of tolerance (25 per cent below target profit) and thus less likely to be able to apply for price increases.

6 Audit Commission, *A Prescription for Improvement*, London: HMSO, 1994, p. 63.

7 Audit Commission, *What the Doctor Ordered*, 1995, p. 32.

8 These are now unitary authorities (known as Health Authorities or Commissions) comprising the old FHSAs together with the former District Health Authorities or DHAs.

9 Audit Commission, *A Prescription for Improvement,* London: HMSO, 1994, p. 62.

10 Burstall, M.C., *1992 and the Regulation of the Pharmaceutical Industry*, Health Series, No. 9, London: IEA Health and Welfare Unit, 1990, p. 78.

11 Boston Consulting Group, *The Changing Environment for US Pharmaceuticals*, Boston, 1993.

Pricing Behaviour, Discounting and Innovations, 1989-95

The Samples and Variables

In each of the six countries over eighty therapeutic sub-markets were examined for the years 1989 through to (September) 1995. The sub-markets (listed in the Appendix) comprised almost the total market, exclusions occurring mainly where sub-markets had products which were non-comparable by presentation, dosage and so also price.

The sub-markets are those devised by the World Health Organisation's (WHO) Anatomic Therapeutic Classification (ATC) system. There are 16 General Groups (e.g. one is Alimentary Tract and Metabolism, another is Systemic Hormones). These are subdivided into 100 Main Groups (so-called second level groupings), and in turn into 284 sub-groups (third level groupings) of which 80 are further divided into 252 fourth level Therapeutic Classes. This study operated at the second level and on occasion at the third. The objective was to work with sub-markets where products would be truly regarded as competing both by prescribers and by manufacturers. That is, a high degree of demand cross-elasticity could be assumed to be present. Or, in less technical language, the products would be regarded as substitutes for each other: if the price of one product rose then more would be bought of the directly competing substitute in the same sub-market and vice versa. Of course products are not necessarily therapeutic substitutes simply because they operate on similar sites in the human body. Conversely, some of the sub-markets regarded as distinct could have been therapeutic substitutes (e.g. cephalosporins are technically different from Broad Spectrum Penicillins yet many would regard them as clinical alternatives—at least on occasion). This arbitrariness imposed on the study by the original database is not, however, serious. First, even if some sub-markets have been inappropriately selected, that inappropriateness applies across all the countries and through each of the seven years examined. General trends (as opposed to levels) of pricing will thus be unaffected. Second, the data are produced by a commercial market research house for resale to commercial firms. If the information and classification system was not useful to competitive decision making it would not be purchased.

The prices of the top five products in each sub-market were found and averaged. "Price" was defined as the price of the top-selling pack size per product. These were frequently in patient-ready packs and so comparable treatment or dosage equivalents. When this was not the case, it tended to be so across the sub-market and hence like was still compared with like. Generally only solid oral presentations were considered (unless all products in the sub-market shared the same presentational form).

Thus annual average sub-market prices were computed unaffected as normal index numbers are by weights relating to volume or values of sales. The aim was to look at prices not index numbers whose values either exaggerate (the Laspeyres index) or understate (the Paasche index) average price movements. Laspeyres or base-weighted indices are computed by taking the prices and volumes sold of a range or 'basket' of products in a base or given year. The index is awarded a value of 100 and compared with some succeeding year's values. The only variables assumed to change are the prices of the original basket of products. Changes in the composition of the basket due to innovation, obsolescence and product improvement are ignored, as are changes in the volumes of the products actually sold. For this reason most medicine price indices published in most countries lag behind the national overall rate of inflation (only the original products have been included). By contrast the same index will overstate the rate of price increase of the basket itself (those older products which have increased in real price will have suffered volume decreases relative to older products whose prices have fallen). The Paasche or current-year index suffers the inverse of these defects. The basket of products selected are those sold today, at today's prices and volumes. A value of 100 is awarded to that basket and compared with the same basket in earlier years assuming again that only the prices, not the volumes, have changed.

In this study the 'basket' was assumed to be the actual top five products sold in the year in question irrespective of sales volumes in other years. The top five products included non-branded generics when recorded. Each average price so computed was then expressed in constant money, adjusting by the inflation rate of the country concerned.

Innovations were priced in the same manner, and were defined as all products new to the sub-market concerned, excluding non-branded generics. The data on innovation, dates of launch, pack size and ex-factory prices were all obtained from Intercontinental Medical Statistics (IMS). The study of innovations was therefore much wider in scope than previous ones (including some done by myself) which were restricted to New Chemical Entities (NCEs). Some of these earlier studies are discussed in Chapter 4 and the results and similarities are contrasted. Most NCEs are not major breakthroughs. This is even more true of other innovations. The question to be answered is not, however, whether innovations have therapeutic value (that is a matter for the clinicians) but rather to assess their economic impact.

The price data IMS present are average prices that pharmacies pay to wholesalers (or directly to manufacturers) for a given dosage, form and strength of a product. The average price is based on a survey of wholesalers, retailers and/or manufacturers' price lists. Because of its data collection methodology, IMS is unable to include rebates, discounts and credits in its calculation price. The IMS data are, therefore, not necessarily accurate estimates of actual transaction prices. This is not a problem if the ratio of the (unknown) actual transaction price to the (known) survey price is constant over time. But if rebates and discounts are increasing or decreasing over time, the IMS data would not capture these changes. As will become apparent there appears to indeed be a trend, in at least two of the countries examined (the USA and South Africa), towards increases in rebates off list prices. That implies that the results presented below will be biased towards under-estimating any actual downward trend in manufacturer's transaction prices discovered in these markets, and conversely, overstating any increases.

The inflation-adjusted average price of the top five products in each sub-market in each country was compared with the preceding year's equivalent figure on a year-on-year basis. The comparison showed average price rises or falls of varying magnitudes. The distribution of these changes in average price is provided in Tables 1A - 1F and is summarised by a straight arithmetic average in Table 1. Figure 1, summarising the data in Table 1, shows that most sub-markets (out of over 480 studied, over 80 per country) continually experienced real year-on-year average price reductions. In Figure 1 only in 1992 did the percentage of sub-markets with real price falls drop below 50 per cent. Figures 1A - 1F and Tables 1A - 1F provide the same data by country. The overall picture is very similar. Sub-markets whose average price level fell outnumbered those experiencing real increases in price. Seven years is a very brief period in which to discern a trend, but Denmark and South Africa appear to be experiencing an increasing number of sub-markets with real price reductions, while in the UK the reverse may be true. In no single year in the UK, however, does the proportion of sub-markets experiencing price increases reach 50 per cent (in 1992 Table 1E identifies just over 40 per cent such sub-markets).The USA has been the most susceptible (in the years under study) to sub-markets displaying price increases. In fact, only in the three years 1993 to 1995 did the proportion of sub-markets with price falls exceed 40 per cent.

The main exceptions are in the countries and years where one-off price reductions were required by government. Thus in Denmark when a one year price freeze was imposed in 1994 (see p. 8 above) the percentage of sub-markets experiencing price rises fell to 28 per cent from 46 per cent in each of 1992 and 1993 (see Table 1A). Similarly (Table 1B, and p. 10 above) when Germany's Health Care Act of 1993 was passed the proportion of sub-markets experiencing price reductions in real terms rose from 42 per cent in 1992 to 66 per cent in 1993. While in the Netherlands (see Table 1C and pp. 10-11 above) the price reductions negotiated in the hope of allowing innovations to be part of the reimbursement process resulted in the proportion of sub-markets with real price reductions—which had averaged 64 per cent in the study period to 1993—peaking at 73 per cent in 1994.

The results are summarised below, but first, six case studies are presented to show how the ebb and flow of rival products affects sub-markets from year to year.

The Case Studies

Case i

Top Five Products and Innovations
Anti-Depressants - South Africa, 1989 Rands

Year	1989	1990	1991	1992	1993	1994	1995
Product							
A	70	72	77	84	77	70	68
B	33	38	38	43	48	44	40
C	35	38	41	41	44	-	-
D	59	60	61	63	69	67	-
E	95	100	101	116	-	-	-
F	-	-	-	-	-	64	66
G	-	-	-	-	77	57	53
H	-	-	-	-	-	-	54
Average	58.4	61.6	63.6	69.4	63.0	60.4	56.2
Innovations							
F			68				
J			21				
G				92			
K						67	
H						57	
I						17	
L						38	
M							53
N							51
O							68
P							29
Average			44.5	92.0		44.8	50.3

The anti-depressant market is a good illustration of innovative rivalry and price competition. Yet it also indicates how difficult it is to observe consistent behaviour merely from the statistics of only one year. The process is complex. Five products dominated the market with no innovations in either 1989 or 1990. Real price rises were observed.

Two innovations (one at a substantial discount) appeared in 1991. Product J never appeared as a major player. Product F was launched at a slight premium and appeared in the top five in 1994 and 1995. Product F fell in price in these years helping to dislodge the higher priced products D and E.

Product G was launched in 1992 at a premium, achieved the top five in 1993 after having been significantly lowered in real price, and continuing to show real price falls in later years. It too helped dislodge the higher priced products D and E.

When innovations appeared in larger numbers in 1994 and 1995, they did so on average at a discount. The price of the top five on average then fell in 1994 and 1995 to a lower level than ruled in 1989.

Case ii
Top Five Products and Innovations
Ace Inhibitors - Denmark, 1989 Kroner

Year	1989	1990	1991	1992	1993	1994	1995
Product							
A	538	544	534	510	504	-	-
B	259	263	257	246	197	197	225
C	554	560	-	-	-	-	-
D	589	-	-	-	-	-	-
E	485	477	467	457	443	433	410
F	-	-	-	-	-	401	384
G	-	547	536	-	-	-	-
H	-	-	489	468	463	452	424
I	-	-	-	316	312	306	289
Average	485	478	456	399	384	358	346
Innovations							
F		352					
E	485						
G	558						
H	513						
I				316			
J		113					
K		603					
L		415					
M		179					
N			243				
O			385				
P					npr		
Q						387	
R						841	
S						384	
T						384	
U							197
V							423
W							218
Average	519	332	314	316	na	499	279

npr = no price recorded

Innovative competition was strong in the Ace inhibitor market. Real prices fell for the top five in the study period (only two of the original five remained in 1995—namely products B and E). Product E was itself an innovation in 1989 entering at a discount to the other three more highly priced leaders. Each of these three dropped out of the top five. From 1990 to 1995 innovations occurred annually. Only in 1994 did the recorded average price of the average innovation fail to be well below the (falling) average price of the top five.

Again, however, although some innovations like product I can be launched at a discount, and bring down top five prices, others like G and H can be introduced at a premium, yet they also contribute to falling prices in the longer term.

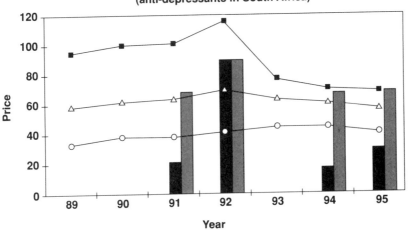

Figure i

Prices of Top 5 Products and Innovations
(anti-depressants in South Africa)

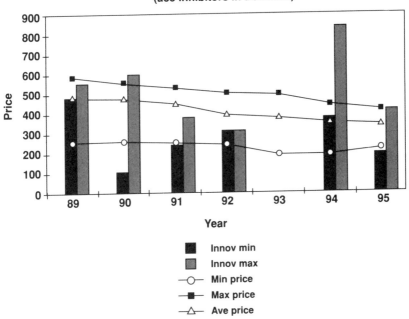

Figure ii

Prices of Top 5 Products and Innovations
(ace inhibitors in Denmark)

Case iii

Top Five Products and Innovations
Tetracyclines and combinations - US
1989 Dollars

Year	1989	1990	1991	1992	1993	1994	1995
Product							
A	93.2	99.9	91	109.2	-	-	-
B	92.6	-	106.3	-	-	-	-
C	-	76.2	76.2	77.5	79.1	-	84.7
D	-	64.0	72.1	76.9	78.7	-	-
E	-	-	51.7	53.0	-	50.7	50.8
F	-	-	-	-	58.2	61.7	63.9
Average	92.87	80.03	82.62	79.13	71.98	56.22	66.48
Innovations							
F				59.5			
Average				59.54			

The tetracycline market is a good example of a technologically mature area with few innovations and a strong presence of non-branded generics. Unidentified generics occupied three of the top five places by sales in 1989 and two in 1995. Technologically the market lies at the opposite extreme to Case (ii) (Ace Inhibitors) where over the study major new products displaced the 1989 top five in 13 situations in later years. In Case (i) (Anti-depressants) the 1989 top five were displaced on only six occasions. Here, due to generics, not to obsolescence, established products entered, left and re-entered the top five. Only two branded products were recorded in the top in 1989 and by 1993 both of these had dropped in sales volume never to reappear among the leaders. But one innovation was recorded in the study period and was launched at a discount. Nevertheless, the rivalry from generics or from that innovation ensured that the price trend was downwards for all years except 1995.

Case iv

Top Five Products and Innovations
Acid Pump Inhibitors - Germany
1989 D Marks

Year	1989	1990	1991	1992	1993	1994	1995
Product							
A	110.1	106.8	102.4	99.1	91.0	87.6	73.6
B	-	106.8	102.4	99.1	91.0	87.8	73.6
C	-	-	-	-	83.8	78.2	68.4
D	-	-	-	-	-	74.9	74.0
E	-	-	-	-	-	74.9	74.0
Average	110.1	106.8	102.4	99.1	88.6	80.7	72.5
Innovations							
B		106.8					
C					83.8		
D						74.9	
E						74.9	
Average		106.8			83.8	74.9	

Acid pump inhibitors is a relatively new market and is very narrowly defined. H2 antagonists, for example are competitors and the impact of their rivalry (or lack of it since it is technologically more mature) is not displayed above. Again the average price in the marketplace fell—by over 30 per cent in real terms. At first—till 1992—reductions were primarily due to the holding steady of money prices. Products C, D and E came in at money discounts, however, so pushing down the real and money prices of products A and B.

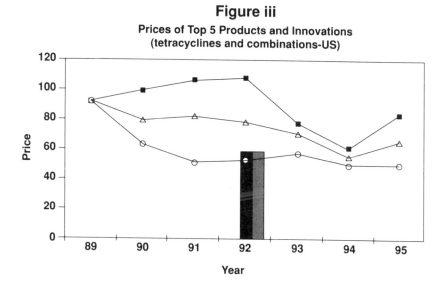

Figure iii

**Prices of Top 5 Products and Innovations
(tetracyclines and combinations-US)**

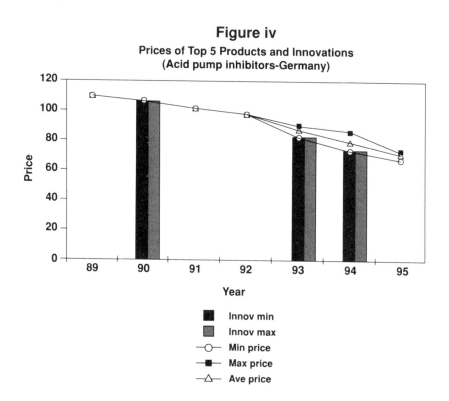

Figure iv

**Prices of Top 5 Products and Innovations
(Acid pump inhibitors-Germany)**

Case v

Top Five Products and Innovations
Fluoroquinolones - UK
1989 pounds

Year	1989	1990	1991	1992	1993	1994	1995
Product							
A13.13	12.08	11.55	11.16	10.9	10.64	10.37	
B 4.73	4.08	1.93	1.86	1.89	-	-	
C25.36	23.35	-	-	21.17	22.11	21.41	
D		11.87	11.35	10.97	13.78	14.42	11.77
E		5.41	5.17	5.00	4.88	4.76	4.65
F			13.46	13.01	-	-	-
Average 14.41	11.36	8.69	8.4	10.52	12.98	12.05	
Innovations							
D		11.87					
E		5.41					
F			13.46				
Average		8.64	13.46				

Fluoroquinolones is occupied by very few products and generics do not achieve a place in the top five. Innovations D and E quickly gained positions in the top five, lowering the market's average price. Product F had a similar effect, albeit introduced at a premium to the average price it temporarily displaced product C in 1991 and 1992. When C regained its position in the top five in 1993 it did so at a lower price than it had held in 1990. Products B and F dropped out of the market completely (not merely the top five) so impacting on the arithmetic average price in 1994, which nonetheless continued downwards from 1994 to 1995. By 1995 the average was well below its 1989 level.

Case vi
Top Five Products and Innovations
Betablocking Agents - Holland 1989 Guilders

Year	1989	1990	1991	1992	1993	1994	1995
Product							
A	18.1	17.3	16.1	15.0	14.7	13.7	13.2
B	18.6	17.7	16.5	15.6	15.3	14.4	13.9
C	63.9	61.2	-	-	-	-	-
D	31.6	-	34.3	39.4	38.5	36.0	-
E	30.9	-	-	-	-	-	-
F	-	29.5	29.1	30.4	29.2	27.8	27.1
G	-	32.0	30.1	29.7	27.1	25.6	25.0
H	-	-	-	-			16.3
Average	32.62	31.5	25.2	26.0	25.0	23.5	19.1
Innovations							
I	29.0	-					
J	31.9	-					
K			15.1				
L			16.8				
M				30.1			
N				19.5			
O						38.7	
P							22.2
Q							18.8
Average	30.5	-	16.0	24.8	-	38.7	20.5

Innovations were frequent in the betablocker market. The average price of the top five fell in all years but one (1992). However, not one innovation succeeded in penetrating the leading ranks. The market turbulence which can be seen from the table was caused entirely by existing products moving into or out of the top five. Products F, G and H all entered the top five but had been launched prior to 1989. All three of these products entered at a price level below the previous year's average. After 1990, C, the highest priced product did not reappear. D, the second highest priced product was dislodged in 1990, reentered in 1991 at a still higher price, and contrary to almost all of the other observations contrived to have its real price increased. It was dislodged again in 1995 by H, an existing product priced below the two innovations of that year, P and Q. Clearly the betablocker innovations failed to have either the price or quality advantage or both which is required successfully to enter the market. Simultaneously, existing products (other than D) were continuously reduced in real price in the face of or because of these innovations, by a sufficient amount, given their clinical qualities, to retain position.

A spot check of other countries in the sample showed that Case vi (for Holland) is not untypical of betablocker markets elsewhere.

Figure v

Prices of Top 5 Products and Innovations
(Fluoroquinolones-UK)

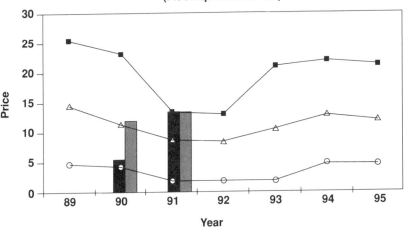

Figure vi

Prices of Top 5 Products and Innovations
(Betablocking agents-Holland)

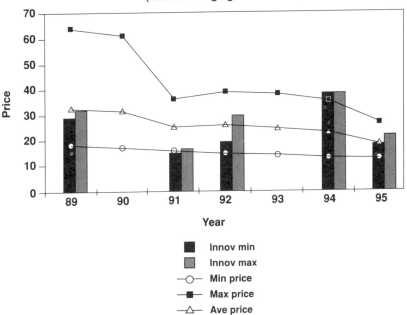

Results

The general result, whether inferred from the main tables or from the cases, is that the majority of sub-markets experience falls in average price in any given year, and that the proportion of such sub-markets is stable in the 50 to 66 per cent range.

Of course this is not the same thing as saying that the overall drug budgets of buyers are falling. First, we are looking at prices unweighted by product volumes. Second, we are examining sub-markets which vary widely in turnover size. Third, we are examining the distribution of these sub-markets by category of average price change. We are not (except in the case studies) following through the average price changes year-by-year of specific sub-markets. Given sub-markets may well form part of the 'price falling' category in one year but part of the 'price rising' category in another year. Fourth, the prices are not necessarily transaction prices after discounts.

Prices fall because of competitive forces and, as the six cases showed, one of the most obvious means of rivalry in pharmaceuticals is from innovative products. There are two difficulties for the observer. One is that innovative competition can be ambiguous. Not all innovations are linked to price competition and, secondly and conversely, not all price rivalry is linked to innovation. Indeed the two effects may be equal and opposite and so cancel out. Indeed this appears to be the implication of Table 2 and the country-by-country Tables 2A - 2F which it partially summarises. The country tables show the number of sub-markets per year which were subject to innovations (out of a total of over 80 sub-markets per annum). The proportion of the sub-markets with innovations experiencing real price changes (up or down) on a year-by-year basis was almost identical to that of all sub-markets (see Table 2). Again it is important to note the caveats of the previous paragraph and not infer from Table 2 more than is claimed. Table 2 is designed not to show why and where drug expenditures are falling, but to show that at first glance the incidence of innovative rivalry on price is not readily apparent.

To tease out the impact of innovations on price reductions Table 3 and Figure 2 were constructed (National Tables 3A-3F and Figures 2A-2F). Column B in Table 3 shows that consistently between two thirds and three quarters of all sub-markets which experienced new product launches saw such innovations being launched at a discount to the ruling average price. Furthermore (column C), over half of the innovations were launched at a discount of over 25 per cent to the ruling average price. In addition, half of the sub-markets which experienced innovations (column D) actually were subject to more than one innovation in a given year. When two or more innovations occurred then the likelihood of discounting was not signifi-cantly, but nonetheless slightly and consistently higher (contrast column E and column B).

Innovations therefore tend to impact downwards on price, either as they themselves move into the top five products or, in reaction to their appearance, existing members of the top five reduce their prices. The majority of sub-markets, therefore, not unsurprisingly consistently display price falls. Again, it is worth referring to the individual cases above for a richer feel of the underlying economic behaviour and confirmation of the general inferences.

However, prices cannot fall everywhere and forever. And they do not. Stable prices in some sub-markets, while others are falling, can simply mean that competition has done or is continuing to do its job. Competition tends to push prices down and to hold them down to a floor. Furthermore, not all innovations are launched at a discount in order to penetrate sub-markets quickly. Some, indeed many—the majority—are. Some of these discounted innovations include major therapeutic advances—priced low perhaps because a similar rival innovation is anticipated to arrive on the marketplace shortly thereafter. Rapid market penetration and fast acquisition of prescriber and patient awareness is then essential if the whole innovative effort on that particular product is not to come to nought.

Table 3, Column B shows that between one third and one quarter of all sub-markets experiencing innovations saw launches being priced at a premium. Some of these products would be major therapeutic advances as discussed in the next paragraph. Many, however, would be of little or minor therapeutic worth in the eyes of the prescribers or patients. Such products tend not to enter the top five (see the Case Studies) and hence have no effect on the average sub-market price computed here. Commercial 'mistakes' of this sort are inevitable, and well documented,[1] and the cost of the error in market judgement is borne by the innovating firm.

Some Implications

Given these harsh economic and competitive realities, some products must successfully generate premium prices in order to maintain the incentives for pharmaceutical advance in health care. These are the relatively rare, or blockbuster, major innovations, which possess a substantial quality increment over existing therapies and so can both command and maintain realistic price premia for reasonable periods. What is required is that sufficiently long periods elapse before the Schumpeterian Gale of Creative Destruction blows. The rewards of innovative profits should not be "washed away" by government induced breaches of intellectual property, whether exercised through weakening of patent protection or by imposition of price controls, or by prescribing limitation or other artificial inhibitions on the commercial marketplace. If innovative profits are encroached on, the incentive to do research for further advances is diluted.[2] Reimbursers, however, need have no concern that they are being exploited. First such premium products are few in number. Grabowski and Vernon have estimated that only 30 per cent of New Chemical Entities (NCEs) cover the average R&D cost of an NCE[3] while only 20 per cent of NCEs provide returns above that level. (And NCEs are a minority of innovations.)

Second, the results from our study show that without any artificial assistance, Schumpeter's competitive gale of innovation, entry, imitation, rivalry and marketplace turbulence is strikingly adequate in its ability to put downward pressure on prices in most markets in most years.

This reasoning and the axiom (although it is not always understood and so accepted as such) that the same prices cannot fall everywhere and always underlies the results. They also again explain why neither base weighted price indices (which tend to undershoot trends in drug expenditures) nor indices using current weights (which overshoot them) capture the full flavour of pharmaceutical rivalry. This needs continuous restatement since the plethora of conflicting and often counter-productive regulations discussed earlier suggest that, even now, the multifaceted real life economics of Schumpeterian innovation are not fully understood by policy makers.

In each market studied competition as a process reduces prices. Innovations are a major part of that competitive process. In the immediate term they can exert a sharp downward jolt to existing price levels. Or, over the longer run, even if, as blockbusters they are introduced initially at higher prices they subsequently reinitiate the downward pressures. Indeed an earlier study showed that even blockbusters are launched at lower prices if firms are aware that the innovation will only have a short competitive lead time. Then pre-emptive low level pricing occurs as the innovator attempts to generate a high market share and so some prescriber loyalty before a similar innovation emerges from the R&D pipeline. (Knowledge of products not yet launched but at late stages of development is widely available to scientists and clinicians working in the field.)[4] Regulation can also reduce prices. And in three countries (Germany, Holland and Denmark) in particular, in identifiable years, our results showing the downward pressure of competitive forces from innovations of all types were exaggerated by regulation induced reductions. Does this suggest it would be desirable to discourage or eliminate by diktat on an *ex ante* basis the commercially inspired innovations which have induced the market turbulence leading to price falls? These suggestions have been made by submissions to both the UK parliament and to the EC (see pp. 1-2 above).

Clearly the answer must be negative. Although in our results the impact of regulation could not be disaggregated from that of competition, it was not that important. The benefits of rivalry, on the other hand were. The benefits of competition, clearly shown in all of the markets studied, would be foregone. Whether the regulations themselves should continue to be encouraged is another matter. What they do is to give some national markets the appearance of more price sensitivity than others.

Firms faced with markets of apparently different price sensitivities will then, if behaving rationally, price more highly (or reduce prices less rapidly) in the more insensitive markets. That rationale explains the

American results in Figure 1F and Table 1F where, contrary to the summary Table 1 and Figure 1, more rises than falls were recorded. But the key result that competition and innovation exerts downward pressure on price is unaffected.

That result, even when modified by rational behaviour in the face of regulation, is not unexpected. It merely broadens understanding of previous studies on the one hand (which tended to be restricted to NCEs) and updates them on the other.

The next Chapter synthesises this study with some earlier ones and draws some broader conclusions.

Notes

1   New product commercial 'failures' are common in many industries. In pharmaceuticals even products deemed important therapeutically by outside observers have failed commercially. When the product is both highly priced and of minor incremental value the chances of failure are even greater. See Reekie, W.D., *Pricing New Pharmaceutical Products*, London: Croom Helm, 1976.

2   Readers unfamiliar with the literature based on the economics of innovation, and in particular the work of Schumpeter, will find a useful introduction with special reference to pharmaceuticals in Teeling-Smith, G., (ed.), *Innovative Competition in Medicine: A Schumpeterian Analysis of the Pharmaceutical Industry and the NHS*, London: Office of Health Economics, 1992.

3   See Reekie, *Prescribing the Price of Pharmaceuticals, op. cit.*, 1995, p. 70.

4   See Reekie, *op. cit.*, 1976, p. 27.

4

Discussion

The results of this study are fully compatible with those carried out either by other investigators or at other times. For example, this author looked at the daily dosage pricing of all NCEs launched in each of the USA, UK and Holland relative to daily dosage costs of existing products in the various therapeutic sub-markets. Major NCEs (as rated by governmental or independent authorities) tended to be introduced at either relatively high prices (often a multiple of existing prices) or, on occasion, at discounted prices if succeeding rivals were anticipated. The less important (incrementally) the NCEs were the lower were their relative prices, until, at a "me-too" level, discounts became common. Further, over time the higher priced innovations fell in price.[1]

A Comparison with Some Previous Studies

These three studies examined every single one of the 120-180 NCEs launched over approximately a decade. A more recent study in the UK examined 84 leader/follower NCEs over 35 years to 1995.[2] The criterion for selecting the 84 was that each was one of a series of at least two NCEs with similar pharmacology. Subsequent NCE launches were introduced at progressively lower prices over the years relative to the lead NCE. By the 1990s these reductions in launch price had bottomed out.

These two groups of studies are consistent with and reinforce each other. They are both in turn compatible with a recent US study over 1991 and 1992 of the launch price levels of 55 drugs approved by the Food and Drug Administration for marketing purposes.[3] Of the 55 only seven were "break-through" drugs where no therapeutic equivalent existed. The remainder (i.e. the great majority) tended to be launched at discounted prices, the discount being greater the greater the likelihood of alternative and approximately similar and equivalent therapies being available. That same study showed that list price increases were moderating over a three-year period and that innovations were linked to that moderation.

The multi-country study reported on in this *Paper* repeats and reinforces these conclusions (albeit from a different starting point in sample design). At any one time more than half of all sub-markets experience price falls, Most sub-markets which experience innovations experience launches occurring at substantial discounts but (inferentially both from the data and from previous studies) premiums are established for innovations where no similar product yet exists. Therefore in such sub-markets prices rise.

This, of course, is not to say that overall price levels—however difficult they are to define given the weighting problems of index numbers—are not changing at a different rate, across countries. For example, reconsider Table 1F, Figure 1F for the USA. In no year did half or more of all sub-markets experience real price falls. Indeed the percentage of markets experiencing increases ranged from 72 per cent in 1991 to a low of 51 per cent in 1994. Irrespective of deficiencies in either index number construction or of the data used in this study, prices in the USA seem generally to have been on an upward trend in that national market. What this study has provided are both international differences in trends and decompositions of these trends with special reference to new product launches.

The economic model which underlies each of the earlier studies was discussed in a recent paper.[4] It need not be restated here. There are, however, implications for price regulators arising from the consensus of the current and past work reported on.

Price competition (modified or enhanced by innovative entry) is strong in the pharmaceutical industry. Study after study over the years has underlined this. That claim does not mean that innovative price rivalry is becoming stronger as two recent studies have claimed. In the US study referred to above a three-year period is an insufficiently long one in which to make such an assertion.[5] In the UK case a 35-year period was used, but the sample drawn examined price ratios of NCEs relative to "break through" prices. This confirmed earlier work. As later incremental advances occur the premium that can be charged for the subsequent new product becomes ever less (where "less" can include discounts in the distribution chain). The longer the time period the greater this process of compression becomes. Any other inference would suggest that either firms in an earlier period were irrationally overpricing or that those in the later years are underpricing (other things equal). Other things, of course, are not equal—for example regulation is ever tougher. Nevertheless, care should be taken not to misinterpret results. If innovation launch prices have fallen, and fallen steadily for nearly 40 years, then taken at face value that suggests lot of irrational (i.e. unremunerative) innovative activity has been occurring for around a generation. A free lunch indeed! The results of that study, however, do not depend on such irrationality. Rather they are simply evidence of ever diminishing incremental therapeutic novelty by NCEs. The more distant in time was the "lead" or "breakthrough" NCE the less incrementally advantageous are subsequent ones, and the declining price ratio uncovered simply reflects this. Block-buster breakthroughs, by definition, were excluded from the data used in that study except (historically) as denominators in a trend of ratios.

Policy Implications

So the problem for policy makers remains. How should innovations, major breakthroughs, with no similar acting existing therapy available, be priced? The UK awards price freedom subject to an overall profit cap. In the US and South Africa, where pluralistic reimbursers exist, individual reimbursers may on occasion, but seldom, refuse reimbursement. Price freedom exists. In reference price countries, some, like Germany, have traditionally immediately reimbursed new products whilst awaiting reference classification. Others, like Holland, are continuing to refuse reimbursement until classification occurs. Still others, like Denmark, "drag feet" in the classification process. Rapid diffusion of innovation is thus discouraged (particularly in the latter two countries). Patients are deprived of the advantages of new therapies, and manufacturers find positive cash flows are pushed into the future, so reducing returns on innovative investments.

The problem, or course, is insoluble for policy makers. The worth of a true innovation (not the costs to the innovator, however defined) is not whether it provides the firm with a return on capital equivalent to the "FT 100" (or any index) but rather what it is worth to the patient in terms of what he or she will willingly pay to acquire its benefits. That can be determined in a free marketplace. Indeed that is the purpose of markets as institutions. But it cannot be determined by a third party in Whitehall or Washington, although a proxy value can be imposed by Whitehall or Washington. The essence is individual choice varying with individual circumstances and knowledge. In practice some, but only some, choosers (patients) can make such a choice individually. In others, agents—third party reimbursers—must make the choice on behalf of patients. A plurality of agents (i.e. reimbursers) is more likely to arrive at a choice close to that of the individual than is some monolithic government agency.

Price studies can only show that competition is working. They cannot evaluate in advance incremental benefits which no consumer has yet judged. The danger is that misinterpretations and misunderstandings result in ever stiffer regulation of innovation. There are no free lunches. In some areas regulation is irrational, and too rigid. In other areas it hampers rather than encourages competition in the marketplace. Thus the continuing and increasing pressure on manufacturers for better price deals in the USA from relatively unregulated distribution channels is evidence of a tougher competitive environment. That tougher environment does not exist in the three reference price countries or in the South African medical scheme market where distribution channels have high costs which may make life tough for consumers or reimbursers but pose little bargaining threat to manufacturers. Deregulation is what is then required of government.

Towards Rational Attitudes To Prices
Pharmaceutical prices are competitively determined. The evidence supports this assertion, so too does the theory. Only the most simplistic of critiques would deny this—namely criticisms based on the use of text book

"perfect" competition as a normative goal. The key point, however, as Hayek put it is not to worry "whether competition in a given case is perfect and worry much more about whether there is competition at all".[6]

Unfortunately, the very existence of price controls (whether of the PPRS variety or reference pricing, or product-by-product controls as exist in some European countries) carries with it the implication that prices are not competitively determined. Historically, after World War II, price regulation in Europe was not confined to pharmaceuticals; controls were pervasive. Gradually in the West they were dismantled until only pharmaceuticals remained under regulation (in the East the dismantling was discrete with the collapse of the command economies). The increasing intensity, not just the continuation, of price controls in pharmaceuticals in Europe has come about as a reaction by governments to the ever increasing costs of paying wholly or partially for health care in a welfare state. This was exacerbated by the fact that once in place, price controls are difficult to remove. A bureaucracy with a vested interest in preserving or enhancing its own career structure jealously guards the system. If the controls fail to achieve their targets, the answer is not to relax them but to apply them more rigorously.

The outcome is to distort the incentives for the supplying industry (and so discourage the innovative activity wanted by consumers). Given international trade, autonomous governments and exchange rate fluctuations, another result of price control is to introduce wasteful anomalies such as parallel importing into the marketplace. This is not to argue, of course, that there should be no pressure for cost containment in pharmaceutical expenditures. The issue is how that pressure should be applied. This returns us full circle to the opening sentences of this section. The alternative to regulation is competition to enable consumers to discuss information about product attributes and, in particular, price; and on product alternatives and, in particular, alternative prices. As Hayek emphasised, prices facilitate informed choice.[7]

"Customers" as decision makers in the health care market include the patient, the doctor-prescriber, the pharmacist-dispenser, and , if present, the third party reimburser, whether state or private insurer. In the two private markets in this study (the USA and South Africa) the development of pressures to cost-contain, to ensure that each element of the "customer" is cost conscious, is becoming ever more sophisticated and effective. PBMs, variable copayments, formularies, generic encouragement, and discounting at all levels of increasingly productive and innovative distribution channels are becoming ever more commonplace. By contrast the NHS has minimal copayments—the prescription charge could be abolished without adverse effect on consumption. It has discouraged disease management and is lukewarm towards PBMs. Whilst the three continental European countries and South Africa protect outmoded and extremely high cost channels of retail distribution.

Not that government reimbursers are ignoring the trend towards controlling the customer (particularly the prescribing component). In fact, in some ways, European governments are controlling customers more than ever before (through positive and negative lists, generic encouragement and indicative prescribing budgets) but they are doing so whilst also further tightening price controls. The ability of the demand side to exert pressure on the supply side (the manufacturers) is, at least in this way, continuously being expanded. The supply side, already behaving competitively, is then further subject to the regulatory pressure of price control with its consequential distortions.

To remove the distortions requires removal of the controls. Removal of the controls would not result in uncompetitive behaviour on the supply side. In all countries examined in this study prices moved competitively.

Schumpeterian innovative competition is pervasive on the supply side. The controls on the demand side, however, do not arise from a plurality of patients and prescribers exerting pressure on suppliers. They are not market pressures reflecting in aggregate individual consumer wants. Rather they are the result of centralised decision taking.

How can government strengthen the demand side further to foster innovative competition? How can it encourage an informed environment rather than a directed one? How can patients and prescribers be empowered so that their individual wishes and wants are responded to by suppliers? Cost conscious consumers will demand cost-effective products and treatments—cost effective, that is, in their eyes, not necessarily in the eyes of the central reimburser.

The tried and tested way, of course, is price. I have already discussed the importance of that issue elsewhere and explained how the existing UK prescription charge could be abolished, bringing a cash nexus between supply and demand closer than it is at present.[8] Copayments are important in each of the countries in this study, and as was noted, only Denmark temporarily and unsuccessfully tried further to exploit their benefits.

Another way of fostering an informed demand side environment, more conducive to innovation than some current controls, is the explicit encouragement of information provision. Thus patients and prescribers could be encouraged to form or associate with groups of patients with common ailments better to understand each others' requirements in order, in turn, more effectively to express and articulate their demands for pharmaceutical therapy. That, in turn, would facilitate the spread of information on what, indeed, is available to the individual patient while prompting suppliers to improve their own individual product offerings. This is no more nor less than a recommendation for sound disease management.

A combination of either price as information, or price with information, will ensure that the views of patients and prescribers are given increasing weight in the marketplace. Suppliers, in turn, will find the pressures

—already present—of Schumpeterian competition will increase as the ever-changing demands of patients for readily available and ever improved medicines become more apparent. And as a corollary, failure to meet such demands will become more transparent, again spurring on the Schumpeterian dynamic.

But so long as the objectives of regulators and reimbursers, on the one hand, and prescribers and patients on the other, do not coincide the tensions will remain. Regulators and reimbursers have budgets and prices as the key components of their utility functions. By contrast, patients and prescribers, like any consumers, achieve satisfaction from consumption (not payment) and from quantities and qualities, and from result. Prices merely assist their choice, and choice exercised provides the ultimate benefit of therapy. Artificial suppression of price by regulators distorts choice. Attempts to discourage innovation by regulation reduces choice. And, by extension, distorted and reduced choice distorts and reduces—in the patient's and prescriber's eyes—the values to them of the ultimate benefit of therapy and cure.

Notes

1   See Reekie, W.D., 'Price and Quality Competition in the United States Drug Industry', *Journal of Industrial Economics*, Vol. 26, No. 3, 1978; Reekie, W.D., (1977) *Pricing New Pharmaceutical Products*, London: Croom Helm, 1977; Reekie, W.D., 'Innovation and Pricing in the Dutch Drug Industry', *Managerial and Decision Economics*, Vol. 1, No. 2, 1982.

2   ABPI, 'Trends in Launch Pricing', Mimeographed, 1996.

3   Boston Consulting Group, *The Changing Environment For US Pharmaceuticals*, Boston, 1993.

4   *Prescribing the Price of Pharmaceuticals, op. cit.*, 1995.

5   *Ibid.*

6   Hayek, F.A., 'The Use of Knowledge in Society', *American Economic Review*, 1945.

7   *Ibid.*

8   *Prescribing the Price of Pharmaceuticals, op. cit.*, 1995.

Appendix
List of Sub-Markets Selected for Study

Plain antacids
H2 Antagonists
Acid pump inhibitors
Plain antispasmodics + Anticholinengerics
Gastroprokinetics
Antiemetic - antinauseants
Protein Lipotropics
Laxatives
Antidiarrhoeals
Antiobesity Preparations
Digestives
Insulin
Oral antidiabetics
Vitamins
Mineral supplements
Tonics
Anabolics systemic
Appetite stimulants
Anticoagulants non-injectable
Platelet Aggregate Inhibitors
Anti-fibronolytics
Antianaemics
Hypolipids/anti-atheroma
Antiarrhythmics
Cardiac stimulants excluding cardiac glycos
Antihypertensives plain central
Antihypertensives plain peripheral
Antihypertensives + diuretics
Rauwolfic alkaloids and antihypertensives
Diuretics
Cerebral + peripheral vaso therapies
Vasoprotectives
Beta blocking agents
Calcium antagonists
Ace inhibitors
Antifungals dermatological
Topical antipruriants
Topical antibiotics antivirals
Topical corticosteroids plain
Topical anti acne preps
Oral anti acne preps
Gynaecological anti-infectives

Sex hormones / systemic action only
Urologicals
Oral corticosteroid plain
Thyroid therapy
Tetracyclines + combinations
Broad spectrum penicillins
Cephalosporins
Trimethopric + similar combinations
Macrolides + similar type
Fluoroquinolones
Medium / Narrow spectrum penicillins
Systemic antifungal agents
Systemic antibacterials
Drugs for tuberculosis
Systemic antivirals
Vaccines
Cytostatics
Cytostatic hormone therapy
Immunostimulating agents
Immunosuppressive agents
Antirheumatics non-steroid plain
Antirheumatics topical
Muscle relaxants, central
Anti-gout preparation
Non-narcotic analgesics
Anti-migraine preps
Anti-epileptics
Anti-Parkinson preps
Neuroleptics
Hypnotics + sedatives
Tranquilizers
Anti-depressants
Psychostimulants
Antiparasitics
Topical nasal preparations
B2-Stimulants inhalants
Xanthines
Non anti-infective cold preparations
Expectorants
Cough sedatives
Antihistamines systemic

Table 1
Six Country Summary
of Year-on-Year Price Changes (%)

Year	1990	1991	1992	1993	1994	1995
% of sub-markets with price changes						
falls of >10%	26	24	20	21	22	19
falls of 5<10%	13	13	7	11	13	10
falls of 0-5%	15	15	19	22	31	30
increases of >0-5%	16	14	16	16	11	15
increases of 5-10%	8	10	9	8	4	5
increases of 10 %	22	24	27	21	19	22

Table 1A
Denmark: Year-on-Year Price Changes (%)

Year	1990	1991	1992	1993	1994	1995
% of sub-markets with price changes						
falls of >10%	13	22	29	33	23	22
falls of 5<10%	8	6	4	9	13	21
falls of 0-5%	9	10	21	12	38	22
increases of >0-5%	28	23	5	10	9	4
increases of >5-10%	18	9	1	3	5	7
increases of 10%	24	33	40	33	14	24
Number of sub-markets	(78)	(79)	(78)	(78)	(78)	(76)

Table 1B
Germany: Year-on-Year Price Changes (%)

Year	1990	1991	1992	1993	1994	1995
% of sub-markets with price changes						
falls of >10%	19	20	15	29	21	15
falls of 5<10%	11	11	6	27	12	8
falls of 0-5%	21	23	21	10	40	30
increases of >0-5%	23	17	23	6	10	24
increases of >5-10%	6	1	7	5	2	5
increases of 10%	21	28	27	7	14	18
Number of sub-markets	(84)	(83)	(84)	(84)	(84)	(84)

Table 1C
Holland: Year-on-Year Price Changes (%)

Year	1990	1991	1992	1993	1994	1995
% of sub-markets with price changes						
falls of >10%	39	34	27	20	32	25
falls of 5<10%	10	8	14	9	18	9
falls of 0-5%	24	19	18	34	23	30
increases of >0-5%	4	4	20	13	6	5
increases of >5-10%	2	8	4	5	1	7
increases of 10%	21	27	17	20	20	25
Number of sub-markets	(82)	(83)	(83)	(82)	(82)	(81)

Table 1D
South Africa: Year-on-Year Price Changes (%)

Year	1990	1991	1992	1993	1994	1995
% of sub-markets with price changes						
falls of >10%	35	20	18	8	18	20
falls of 5<10%	4	9	4	5	17	7
falls of 0-5%	9	16	7	7	30	33
increases of >0-5%	10	15	35	30	7	17
increases of >5-10%	4	10	15	23	5	4
increases of 10%	39	31	21	27	24	19
Number of sub-markets	(81)	(81)	(84)	(84	(84)	(84)

Table 1E
United Kingdom: Year-on-Year Price Changes (%)

Year	1990	1991	1992	1993	1994	1995
% of sub-markets with price changes						
falls of >10%	32	32	15	15	18	10
falls of 5<10%	43	40	12	8	12	8
falls of 0-5%	9	11	32	40	34	47
increases of >0-5%	5	5	13	13	14	12
increases of 5-10%	4	4	6	6	4	2
increases of 10 %	9	9	21	17	18	20
Number of sub-markets	(82)	(82)	(84)	(84)	(83)	(83)

Table 1F
USA: Year-on-Year Price Changes (%)

Year	1990	1991	1992	1993	1994	1995
% of sub-markets with price changes						
falls of >10%	19	17	16	21	21	20
falls of 5<10%	1	1	4	7	6	6
falls of 0-5%	20	10	12	19	21	18
increases of >0-5%	27	10	12	25	19	29
increases of >5-10%	12	27	19	7	7	4
increases of 10%	20	35	37	20	25	24
Number of sub-markets	(83)	(82)	(83)	(84)	(84)	(84)

Table 2
Six Country Summary
(Sub-markets subject to Price Reductions)

Year	Percentage of Sub-markets Subject to Real Price Reduction[ii]	Percentage of Sub-markets with Innovations Subject to Price Reductions[iii]
1990	54	55
1991	52	54
1992	46	42
1993	52	51
1994	66	66
1995[i]	59	53

i   9 months only
ii   source table 1
iii   source tables 2A-2F

Table 2A
Denmark: Sub-markets with Innovations by Price Change Category

Year	1990	1991	1992	1993	1994	1995
% of sub-markets with innovations						
falls of >10%	14	17	28	39	21	8
falls of 5<10%	17	3	4	1	18	17
falls of 0-5%	7	9	8	4	36	25
increases of >0-5%	21	31	4	-	4	-
increases of >5-10%	17	9	4	1	4	17
increases of 10%	24	31	52	15	18	33
Number of sub-markets	(29)	(34)	(25)	(29)	(28)	(12)

Table 2B
Germany: Sub-markets with Innovations by Price Change Category

Year	1990	1991	1992	1993	1994	1995
% of sub-markets with price changes						
falls of >10%	19	25	16	33	19	15
falls of 5<10%	14	9	6	29	18	12
falls of 0-5%	24	29	27	13	40	29
increases of >0-5%	22	18	18	10	9	24
increases of >5-10%	3	2	6	6	2	3
increases of 10%	17	18	27	10	12	18
Number of sub-markets	(57)	(56)	(49)	(52)	(57)	(34)

Table 2C
Holland: Sub-markets with Innovations by Price Change Category

Year	1990	1991	1992	1993	1994	1995
% of sub-markets with innovations						
falls of >10%	42	31	22	14	21	18
falls of 5<10%	13	7	7	18	16	27
falls of 0-5%	17	33	11	23	26	18
increases of >0-5%	4	-	33	18	11	-
increases of >5-10%	4	7	7	5	-	18
increases of 10%	21	31	19	23	26	18
Number of sub-markets	(24)	(29)	(27)	(22)	(18)	(11)

Table 2D
South Africa: Sub-markets with Innovations by Price Change Category

Year	1990	1991	1992	1993	1994	1995
% of sub-markets with price changes						
falls of >10%	35	33	17	11	19	21
falls of 5<10%	-	3	9	2	13	8
falls of 0-5%	9	8	6	9	33	38
increases of >0-5%	9	14	23	30	4	21
increases of >5-10%	6	3	17	14	8	4
increases of 10%	41	39	29	34	23	8
Number of sub-markets	(34)	(36)	(34)	(44)	(48)	(23)

Table 2E
United Kingdom: Sub-markets with Innovations by Price Change Category

Year	1990	1991	1992	1993	1994	1995
% of sub-markets with price changes						
falls of >10%	43	31	17	14	25	9
falls of 5<10%	33	43	14	14	8	9
falls of 0-5%	13	11	21	36	38	45
falls of >0-5%	0	9	17	11	8	36
increases of >5-10%	3	3	7	8	8	-
increases of 10%	7	3	24	17	13	-
Number of sub-markets	(30)	(35)	(29)	(36)	(24)	(11)

Table 2F
USA: Sub-markets with innovations by Price Change Category

Year	1990	1991	1992	1993	1994	1995
% of sub-markets with price changes						
falls of >10%	16	18	18	23	20	12
falls of 5<10%	3	0	3	8	9	6
falls of 0-5%	13	15	18	15	18	18
increases of >0-5%	32	12	11	26	16	36
increases of >5-10%	13	18	11	8	11	6
increases of 10%	24	38	39	21	27	21
Number of sub-markets	(37)	(34)	(38)	(39)	(45)	(33)

Table 3
Six Country[i] Summary
of Innovative Pricing Levels

Year	A Sub-markets with innovations	B[ii] % of sub-markets where innovations were launched at a discount	C % of sub-markets where discount exceeded 25%	D % of sub-markets with more than one innovation	E % of column D where innovations were launched at a discount
1989	212	73	54	52	76
1990	211	69	49	55	76
1991	226	65	51	53	68
1992	202	70	54	52	73
1993	222	63	48	48	69
1994	221	63	51	57	69
1995[iii]	127	75	61	36	77

i USA, UK, Germany, South Africa, Holland and Denmark
ii the average innovation price was below the average price of the leading five products in the relevant sub-market.
iii first nine months only

Table 3A
Denmark

Year	A Sub-markets with innovations	B % of sub-markets where innovations were launched at a discount	C % of sub-markets where discount exceeded 25%	D % of sub-markets with more than one innovation	E % of column D where innovations were launched at a discount
1989	30	60	37	37	55
1990	29	69	34	38	83
1991	34	50	41	44	47
1992	25	60	36	48	58
1993	29	62	38	41	75
1994	28	50	39	36	50
1995	12	75	67	8	100

Table 3B
Germany

Year	A Sub-markets with innovations	B % of sub-markets where innovations were launched at a discount	C % of sub-markets where discount exceeded 25%	D % of sub-markets with more than one innovation	E % of column D where innovations were launched at a discount
1989	60	82	75	75	89
1990	57	75	53	81	76
1991	56	75	55	73	78
1992	49	80	67	73	81
1993	52	73	60	65	74
1994	57	74	58	77	73
1995	34	63	59	44	73

Table 3C
Holland

Year	A Sub-markets with innovations	B % of sub-markets where innovations were launched at a discount	C % of sub-markets where discount exceeded 25%	D % of sub-markets with more than one innovation	E % of column D where innovations were launched at a discount
1989	28	50	32	43	33
1990	24	50	29	25	17
1991	29	66	59	34	70
1992	27	56	44	33	44
1993	22	50	27	18	50
1994	19	42	37	16	33
1995	11	73	36	18	50

Table 3D
South Africa

Year	A Sub-markets with innovations	B % of sub-markets where innovations were launched at a discount	C % of sub-markets where discount exceeded 25%	D % of sub-markets with more than one innovation	E % of column D where innovations were launched at a discount
1989	23	87	48	39	89
1990	34	62	50	38	62
1991	38	66	58	45	71
1992	34	65	47	44	80
1993	44	59	48	61	63
1994	48	63	42	63	70
1995	25	72	40	36	67

58

Table 3E
United Kingdom

Year	A Sub-markets with innovations	B % of sub-markets where innovations were launched at a discount	C % of sub-markets where discount exceeded 25%	D % of sub-markets with more than one innovation	E % of column D where innovations were launched at a discount
1989	33	70	42	45	73
1990	30	60	47	40	92
1991	35	60	43	43	53
1992	29	66	55	34	40
1993	36	58	39	31	73
1994	24	54	46	42	50
1995	11	73	73	18	50

Table 3F
Unites States of America

Year	A Sub-markets with innovations	B % of sub-markets where innovations were launched at a discount	C % of sub-markets where discount exceeded 25%	D % of sub-markets with more than one innovation	E % of column D where innovations were launched at a discount
1989	38	79	66	47	87
1990	37	86	68	73	85
1991	34	65	50	65	67
1992	38	79	61	63	88
1993	39	67	59	46	67
1994	45	73	67	64	79
1995	34	85	79	50	88

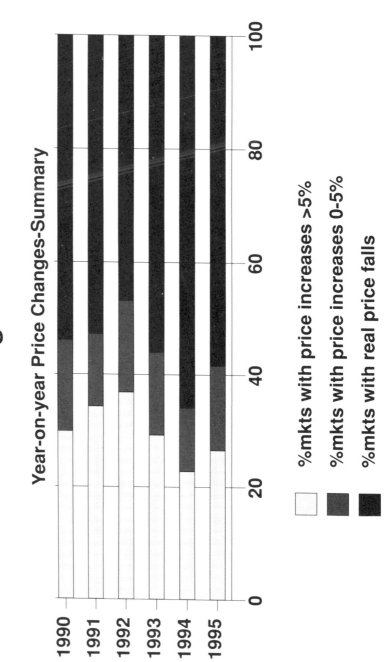

Figure 1

Year-on-year Price Changes-Summary

□ %mkts with price increases >5%

▨ %mkts with price increases 0-5%

■ %mkts with real price falls

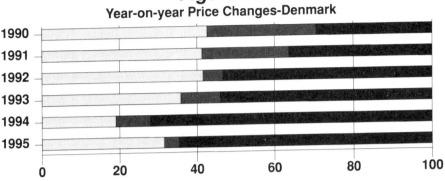

Figure 1a
Year-on-year Price Changes-Denmark

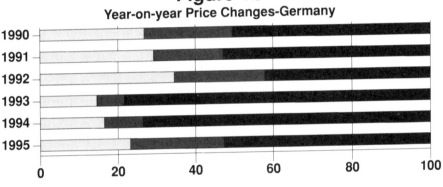

Figure 1b
Year-on-year Price Changes-Germany

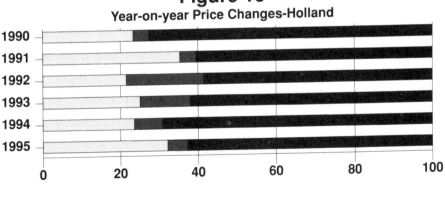

Figure 1c
Year-on-year Price Changes-Holland

%mkts with price increases >5%

%mkts with price increases 0-5%

%mkts with real price falls

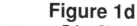

Figure 1d
Year-on-year Price Changes-S Africa

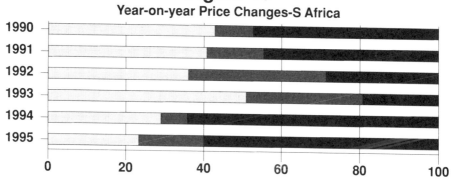

Figure 1e
Year-on-year Price Changes UK

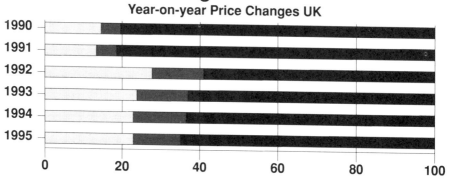

Figure 1f
Year-on-year Price Changes-USA

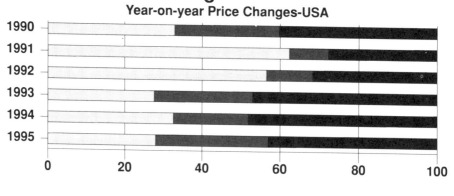

☐ %mkts with price increases >5%

■ %mkts with price increases 0-5%

■ %mkts with real price falls

63

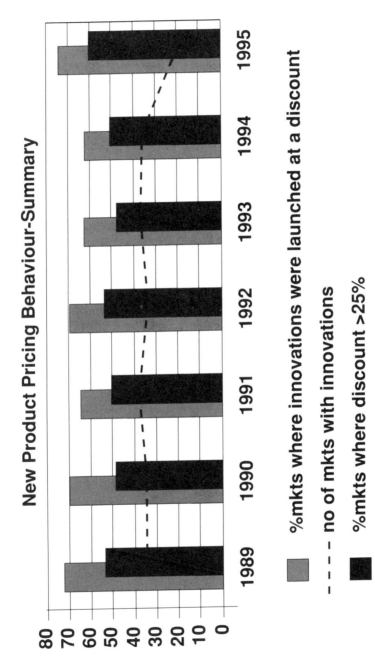

Figure 2

New Product Pricing Behaviour-Summary

Figure 2a

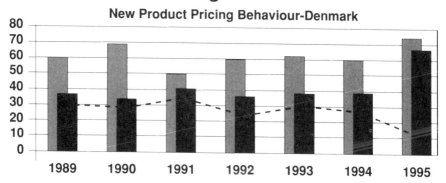

New Product Pricing Behaviour-Denmark

Figure 2b

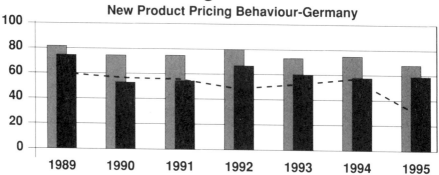

New Product Pricing Behaviour-Germany

Figure 2c

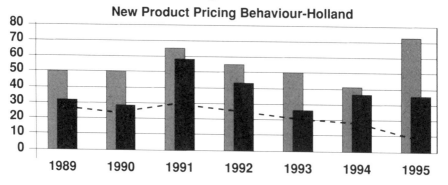

New Product Pricing Behaviour-Holland

%mkts where innovations were launched at a discount
- - - - no of mkts with innovations
%mkts where discount >25%

Figure 2d

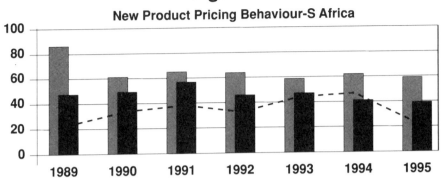

Figure 2e

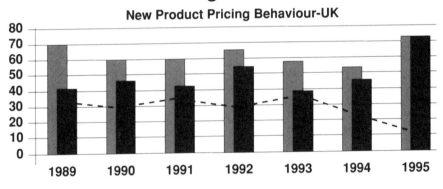

Figure 2f

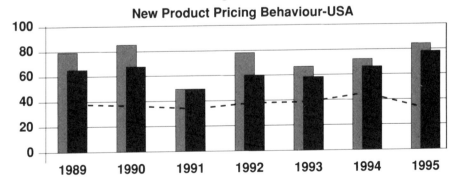